Biology and emotion

Problems in the Behavioural Sciences

Biology and emotion

Neil McNaughton

Department of Psychology
Otago University
Dunedin, NZ

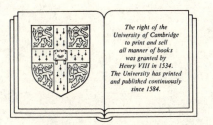

The right of the
University of Cambridge
to print and sell
all manner of books
was granted by
Henry VIII in 1534.
The University has printed
and published continuously
since 1584.

CAMBRIDGE UNIVERSITY PRESS

Cambridge

New York Port Chester

Melbourne Sydney

Published by the Press Syndicate of the University of Cambridge
The Pitt Building, Trumpington Street, Cambridge CB2 1RP
32 East 57th Street, New York NY 10022, USA
10 Stamford Road, Oakleigh, Melbourne 3166, Australia

First Published 1989

Printed in Great Britain at the University Press, Cambridge

British Library cataloguing in publication data
McNaughton, N.
Biology and emotion – (Problems in the behavioural sciences, 5)
1. Man. Emotions, Psychophysiological aspects.
I. Title
152.4

Library of Congress cataloguing in publication data
McNaughton, N.
Biology and emotion
(Problems in the behavioural sciences)
Bibliography: p.
Includes Index.
1. Emotions – Physiological aspects. 2. Emotions. 3. Evolution. I. Title.
II. Series [DNLM: 1. Biology. 2. Emotions. BF 531 M478b]
QP401.M36 1989 152.4 88-22850

ISBN 0 521 26527 4 hard covers
ISBN 0 521 31938 2 paperback

To Julie

La Coeur a ses raisons que la raison ne connaît point
Emotion has its own reasons about which reason knows nothing at all

Blaise Pascal: Pensées (iv, 277 – Brunschvicg)

Contents

Preface

The impetus for this book came when I was delivering a series of undergraduate lectures on emotion to psychology students at the University of Oxford. I was unable to find what I considered a suitable basic text for the course. The available books consisted almost entirely of presentations of particular theories of emotion. It struck me as strange that any field of science should have such a multiplicity of theories – except for the fact that in many cases different theorists were addressing different data bases. What seemed to me to be lacking, therefore, was a general pretheoretical framework into which all of the relevant data could be fitted.

This book is an attempt to provide such a framework. It does not present a specific theory of emotion, although it might bias one in favour of some theories rather than others. The central idea of the book is that biology and particularly evolution provide the best starting point for the study of emotion. This idea is neither novel, since it is the basis for Darwin's work, nor is it unrepresented in current theorising (see particularly Plutchik's various works). However, I do not think its implications have ever been considered outside the bounds of specific theorising. In particular, I have tried to show that all of the conventional properties of emotion such as expression, feeling, and motivation can be considered in a scientific manner and useful conclusions drawn therefrom. For some reason the study of emotion, even now, is bedevilled by reports which are remarkably poor from a scientific and particularly a biological point of view – even when their statistical expertise and basic experimental design are formally correct.

It should be emphasised that the book is not intended as a comprehensive review of any of the areas of emotion it covers. This would have required a much larger book, and the inclusion of general review material would have obscured the central theme. Specific aspects of emotion have usually been discussed only in terms of a limited number of emotions. However, in discussing the different aspects of emotion I have attempted to cover a range of emotions. I hope that the general approach taken in the book will safely allow expansion of the ideas to other emotions to be left as 'an exercise for the student'. While it does not have the usual form of a text, and is not intended primarily as one, I hope the book has been written clearly enough to be useful to undergraduates. I have, myself, used parts of it as the basis for a second year undergraduate course.

In Chapter 1 I discuss the problems which arise from the lack of a satisfactory definition of emotion in psychology. I suggest that a biological and particularly an evolutionary approach to the subject can circumvent many of the problems of definition. I then describe briefly some of the historical approaches to emotion which have led to the modern areas of research reviewed in later chapters. In this context, I should comment on two specific omissions from the book of what might be thought appropriate to the analysis of biological aspects of emotion. The first is the work of Freud. It can be argued that Freud has made a major contribution to the theoretical analysis of emotion. However, the book as a whole attempts to avoid theory and, in particular, Freud's work does not appear to me to provide the foundation for any distinct and fruitful area of modern objective data collection. The second omission is that of essentially neurophysiological theories (e.g. Papez, 1937; Pribram, 1970) and data. This is not because analysis of brain mechanisms is not relevant to emotion, but because it is necessary to decide, via psychology, what are the important elements of a behavioural system before neurophysiology and anatomy can take one very far. Chapter 2 deals with some highly selected neurophysiological observations which help to clarify basic issues. However, a proper physiological analysis of the behavioural systems discussed here would require several additional volumes.

The central points derived from the brief discussion of brain mechanisms in Chapter 2 are: 1) that effector programs (that is to say, integrated responses of glandular, autonomic, or motor system – including facial expressions and directed actions) can be viewed as being released (or triggered) by internal or environmental stimuli; and 2) that certain states of the organism can be viewed as enabling a range of different effector programs rather than unconditionally producing a specific one. The innate elements of such programs would be subject to selection pressure, and, in Chapter 3, I develop the suggestion that a useful *working* definition of specific emotions can be arrived at by considering the coincident evolutionary pressures that may have shaped the control of the various components of emotional reactions. The advantage of such a working definition is that it does not prejudge either a final definition of any particular emotion, or the question of whether different components of emotional reaction share a common central controlling state.

In Chapters 4, 5 and 6 I discuss the form of emotional expression provided by systems designed to communicate between individuals (particularly those controlling facial expression) and those provided by autonomic and hormonal systems which can be seen as systems which communicate between mental state and basic physiological systems. The innate aspects of the systems, viewed as clusters of released reactions, are emphasised in these chapters and the way in which they could have evolved is discussed. It is argued that, in many cases, what are now important reactions psychologically have their origins in reactions which originally evolved in response to basic physiological selection pressures. In Chapter 7 I consider in depth an example of the type of psychological factor which could exert pressure on a pre-existing physiological reaction and emphasise the difference between the nature of the selection pressure, for which a theorist may be able to discern some optimal adaptive strategy, and the number and variety of 'rule of thumb' mechanistic strategies which may concurrently satisfy that selection pressure.

In Chapters 8 and 9 I consider the role of development and learning in emotion as an antidote to the idea that the innate basis of emotional reactions could mean that the form of such reactions in adults is rigidly fixed. In Chapter 9 I consider in particular the status of emotion within learning theory and argue that emotion and motivation should be seen as discrete entities. I also suggest that the methods of the 'behaviour analysts' are particularly suited to the analysis of cognitive strategies in differing species and to the analysis of the extent to which we can validly refer to central states of the animal when discussing emotion.

In Chapter 10 I describe a number of interactions between expressive, autonomic, hormonal, directed skeletal (motor), and cognitive systems in emotion. These had been considered in isolation in previous chapters. I conclude that there may be sufficient interaction between the different components of emotion to justify the use of specific emotion labels, but that control of those components by some single central state remains to be demonstrated for specific emotions.

In Chapter 11 I discuss the vexed question of how far results from one species can be generalised to others. While I acknowledge that each individual species is unique, I conclude that there is no reason to treat humans, within biology, in a different way from any other species.

In Chapter 12 I discuss the application of the ideas presented in the earlier chapters – with particular reference to the dangers of too hasty an attempt to provide an explanation of emotion. The tendency of theorists to dichotomise continua (e.g. nature–nurture) is a particular problem in this area. My final conclusion is that an attempt to achieve an exact definition of emotion, in general, or of any specific emotion, in particular, is premature. However, a biological approach can allow integration of data and can frame valid experimental questions about emotion, even in the absence of such definitions.

This book covers a wide range of topics. In attempting to cover them without making too many blunders, I have sought criticism from a number of colleagues and have benefited from casual discussion of the issues raised in the book with many more. It is usual to absolve one's colleagues from any responsibility for the material in the text. This is particularly necessary in the present case since I was frequently helped by those who specifically disavowed any agreement with my conclusions, while being lavish in their advice as to how better to present the arguments for them.

Acknowledgements

During the writing of this book I have enjoyed the stimulating atmosphere provided by my colleagues in the Department of Psychology at the University of Otago. Whatever the topic under discussion, their enthusiasm for the scientific approach to psychology has encouraged me in my work. Of those whose discussion directly contributed to this book, I owe a particular debt to Graham Goddard. His steadfast refusal to believe that 'emotion' was a topic which had any place in modern psychology bolstered my resolve to complete the book and affected the level at which I pitched a number of the arguments. His contribution to the central ideas of the book – the 'state dependent reflex' – can be judged by the reader. The invigorating departmental atmosphere at Otago is a direct result of his efforts as chairman of the department. His recent tragic death in a tramping accident is a loss both to his department and to the scientific community at large. I hope that this book and other scholarly work from the department in the future will act as a fitting memorial to him.

A number of people read drafts of specific chapters: Cliff Abraham, Derek Blackman, Mike Davison, Louis Leland, Gay Maxwel, Mel Pipe and Gill Rhodes. Chris Linsell and Ed Kairiss both read the entirety of the first draft. All of them offered most useful advice and suggested many modifications and corrections. Many undergraduates taking my course on biology and emotion at Otago have offered specific advice and criticism. I have also been fortunate in my editor, Jeffrey Gray. His capacity for informed disagreement during my years at Oxford shaped many of the ideas which ultimately led to this volume; and his diagnosis of the ills which afflicted the first draft played a major part in the present form of the book. Julie McNaughton read the entire book and offered considerable literary advice which I have attempted to follow. Any clarity of expression the book may have is owed to her. Euan McNaughton generously provided many first-hand data which considerably influenced my views on the development of emotion in the neonate.

1:   Emotion since Darwin

'When I use a word,' Humpty Dumpty said in a rather scornful tone, 'It means just what I choose it to mean – neither more nor less.'

'The question is,' said Alice, 'whether you *can* make words mean so many different things.'

'The question is,' said Humpty Dumpty, 'which is to be Master – that's all.'

Lewis Carroll: Through the Looking Glass

1.1.   What is an emotion?

Emotion is a striking feature of human experience. In any one day we may experience fear, love, pity, rage and many more. Emotion colours our everyday thoughts and actions and generates most of the behaviour which makes our friends and neighbours interesting. Much of Art and Literature is devoted to exploring its subtleties and, at a more practical level, emotions sway events in politics and commerce to a frightening extent. Psychology, the science of the mind, might therefore be expected to give pride of place to emotion as a topic of concern.

Unfortunately, there has never been any clear agreement as to what the word means. Amongst philosophers, 'emotion has almost always played an inferior role ... often as an antagonist to logic and reason ... Along with this general demeaning of emotion in philosophy comes either a wholesale neglect or at least retail distortion in the analysis of emotions' (Solomon, 1977, cited by Lyons, 1980, p ix). Psychologists have followed this lead. Those who are sure that they know the meaning of the word emotion have often proceeded to experiment without ensuring that what they wish to study is objectively identifiable. Those who are unsure as to its meaning have often attempted to solve the problem by purely linguistic analysis without recourse to experimental data at all. More frequently work on emotion has been avoided altogether since it is viewed as disreputable and unscientific. Some texts on learning (Kimble, 1961; Mackintosh, 1974), cognition (Neisser, 1967; Wickelgren, 1979) and even general psychology (Isaacson, Hutt, & Blum, 1965) have no mention of 'emotion' in either chapter headings or index.

So, should we follow the psychologists and throw away any idea of emotion? Are there no objectively identifiable phenomena to which

1

the word can refer? Or, are the psychologists glossing over some important aspect of the control of behaviour? Certainly, the texts I have cited not only do not use the term 'emotion', they also mention only in passing many phenomena which could relate to emotion. This suggests that they may be avoiding the issue. On the other hand the colloquial use of a single word to refer to some item is no guarantee that the item is simple in structure, function or any other attribute.

The lack of an acceptable theory of emotion does not stem from a paucity of candidates (a smorgasbord of these is served in Strongman, 1978). Many books have been written presenting this or that theory of emotion. However, most have a selective view of observational and experimental evidence, often omitting whole areas of research which another theorist would deem pertinent. Both this disparity of viewpoint between theorists and the logical confusion which can be found within some theories are traceable to variations in the meaning of the word emotion. The response of philosophers to this situation is reminiscent of someone walking on tiptoe through a mine field. For example, one 'causal–evaluative theory of emotions' proceeds from the following propositions:

1. That this account is of occurrent emotional states rather than of emotions considered dispositionally;
2. That the concept of emotion as occurrent state involves reference to an evaluation which causes abnormal physiological changes in the subject of the evaluation;
3. That it is by means of the evaluative aspect that we differentiate the emotions;
4. That the concept of particular emotional states may include desires as well as evaluations and physiological changes;
5. That the central evaluative aspect gives rise to emotional behaviour via a rational, and causal, link with desires;
6. That making evaluation to be central to emotion does not mean that emotions are intangible and non-objective.

(Lyons, 1980, p.53)

To the person who wants to know why we cry or why we smile, a preamble such as this does not hold out much hope for a simple, comprehensible answer. (Note, for example, that frequently occurring, and hence presumably 'normal' emotions are defined in terms of 'abnormal' physiological change!) However, the philosopher's somewhat tentative approach appears less unreasonable if we remember the tricks language can play on the unwary scientist.

First, our definition of a word may be ambiguous. It is clearly going to cause problems if, without warning, the same word can refer to two entirely separate entities, e.g. 'vest' – in America, this is worn over the shirt, and in Britain, under it.

Secondly, even a clear unambiguous word may refer to a nonexistent entity, e.g. 'Unicorn'.

Thirdly, a clear objective (even ostensive) distinction may have no counterpart in physical scientific analysis. Consider our ideas of colour: we talk as if there are many identifiable, perceivably different, colours and we can usually agree as to the colour of any particular object. But, from the point of view of a physicist, colour derives from an electromagnetic continuum in which there are no discrete boundaries and of which large portions cannot be seen with the naked eye. Equally, from the point of view of a psychologist, or the designer of a colour television set, our perception of the full range of colours requires the reception of only three different wavelengths of light and many colours may need only two (Land, 1959).

Fourthly, a clear, well-understood scientific concept may cut across discrete categories accepted by language. An electron can be thought of as a particle, a wave, both or neither. From the point of view of the English language, waves must travel in a medium while particles cannot have a wavelength. Neither of these restrictions bothers the physicists – who are quite happy to calculate the wavelength of an elephant.

Fifthly, it may take considerable effort to determine what is normally meant by a word such as emotion and there may be considerable variation in the answer to this question among different people (Davitz, 1969).

These linguistic problems suggest that we could gain by avoiding undue dependence on the specific content of our language. We would not, then, have to discover by experimental or philosophical analysis the exact meaning or meanings of 'emotion' as it is used in everyday speech. None the less, it is useful, by way of a starting point, to look briefly at the question 'What is an emotion?'. This question has bedevilled psychologists since William James asked it in 1884. It appears to invite us to lift ourselves up by our own bootstraps. If we cannot agree on the meaning of the word, how can we use it objectively? But, if we do not use it, how can we refer to the phenomena which we wish to study? Taken in this narrow way 'What is an emotion?' is a pseudoquestion or at least a diversion. It invites us to answer a scientific question before we have collected the data on which the answer should properly be based; or it invites us to confuse a semantic or metaphysical question with a scientific one. As Mandler (1975) points out 'it seems useful not to fall into the trap of trying to explain what "emotion" is; ...

instead [we should describe] a system that has as its product some of the observations that have been called "emotion" ... But the eventual aim is psychological theory not an analysis of human experience expressed in phenomenal, existential or ordinary language.'

One way to proceed, therefore, is as follows. We allow any and every meaning of the word emotion (without worrying about the exact nature of the meanings) to outline an approximate area of observation and experiment. We then attempt to account for as much of the data as possible with some small number of assumptions. Some part of the resultant theory may then be found to map back to our original conception of emotion, providing a scientific definition of the term. On the other hand, it may not, in which case our answer to the question 'What is an emotion?' is that scientifically speaking there is no such thing (Duffy, 1941; 1962). I would probably not have written this book if I believed this last to be likely. However, the book does not pretend to resolve the issue; it does not purvey a new wonder theory of emotion; rather, it attempts to provide a solid base for the further scientific analysis of emotional phenomena.

The list of emotions shows that phenomena related to them will be very numerous. It includes: love, pity, hate, rage, frustration, fear, grief, despair, joy and many others. In addition, the colloquial use of these concepts implies a number of different aspects, including at least:

1. communication – 'he gave me a scared look';
2. feeling – you 'feel' afraid, tremble with fear, go cold with fear;
3. physiological response – 'I broke into a cold sweat', 'my heart was pounding';
4. motivation – fear of the lion will be accompanied by a strong tendency to remove yourself from its vicinity;
5. cognition – we usually know what we are afraid of.

This conceptual richness creates a problem. If we use colloquial terms solely to delineate the area of study, and if we exclude them from our initial analysis of the data, how are we to organise the data so that we are not overwhelmed with detail? Existing theories of emotion, just as much as everday language, are laden with assumptions and different meanings of the critical terms. To use them runs the risk of undervaluing data which, while peripheral to the theories, can provide a bridging link between the areas of data from which the different theories are derived. What is required is some pretheoretical means of organising the data so that analysis can be restricted to coherent subsets of the available facts.

1.2.   A biological approach to emotion?

Some concept such as emotion is explicit or implicit in a wide variety of areas of psychological research. While 'emotion' may be taken to imply a complex internal or mental state, it has proved more parsimonious to treat emotions within psychology as potential intervening variables or theoretical constructs (Brown & Farber, 1951; Goldstein, 1968). We can take a more complicated position when the data force us to it. Brown & Farber make the point that 'emotion may be retained as a separate construct if, and only if, it is empirically useful to posit a state or process that is related to antecedent events, to other constructs, or to behaviour by a different set of functions from those that characterise other constructs within a theory'. A major question in what follows will be how far such intervening variables (states/processes) in one area of research, whether labelled as emotions or not, can be identified with similar intervening variables in other areas.

This question is particularly appropriate at the present time. Many of the areas which touch on emotion are moving together: learning theorists are employing theoretical constructs which border on the cognitive (Dickinson, 1980); physiological psychologists are attempting to relate their work to both learning theory (Gray, 1982) and cognitive psychology (O'Keefe & Nadel, 1978); and the boundaries between ethology, neurophysiology, and the experimental analysis of behaviour are becoming blurred (Masterson & Crawford, 1982; Konishi, 1971; Shettleworth & Juergensen, 1980; McFarland, 1971). Similarly, recent anthologies of work on emotion have covered a wide range of research areas (Rorty, 1980; Arnold, 1970; Izard, 1979) as have recent textbooks (e.g. Buck, 1976). It is clear that areas such as ethology, physiological psychology, psychophysiology, neuropsychology, learning theory, social psychology and cognitive psychology can all shed light on the nature of emotion. I hope this book will also convince you that the study of emotion requires an integration of these areas which, in turn, sheds light on them.

A brief glance at these areas of research suggests a way out of the impasse generated by the slippery nature of the word emotion. Analysis of the expression of the emotions, physiological changes during emotion, the development of emotional behaviour and the incursion of terms related to emotion into theories of learning all imply that emotions, in humans and other animals, are dependent to a considerable extent on aspects of mind/behaviour which are both functionally fundamental and phylogenetically old. A biological approach is likely, therefore, to provide a good starting point for the analysis of emotions.

There are two immediate consequences of such an approach. First, it necessitates a concentration on reliable observation and experimental data which can bypass much of the linguistic confusion which arises when dealing with emotion. Second, it provides a means of compartmentalising the data, and hence dealing with it piecemeal. Functionally discrete systems can be separately analysed, and the different potential components of emotional responses (physiological, expressive, etc.) can be compared to equivalent non-emotional responses.

Note that I am suggesting only that biology (viewed here as the incursion of evolutionary, physiological, and similar considerations into psychology) provides a good starting point. While this book is largely biological in its approach to emotional concepts, the study of emotion properly extends to other disciplines (for example, clinical, cognitive and social psychology). It is my contention that the framework developed in this book provides a sound foundation on which such disciplines can build. It is also my view that the more complex human emotions will only be properly analysed when we have a good understanding of more basic emotions – it is even possible that much of what is viewed as complex and uniquely human may be explicable solely in terms of such simpler emotions.

Not only may 'complex' emotions be constructed from the same, or similar, elements as 'simple' ones, but any individual emotion can be investigated at a number of levels. Suppose we have been asked a question such as 'Why do we cry?'. The answer to this will depend on the context of the question. We could be concerned with social/historical reasons for crying; individual/developmental reasons; psychological processes; physiological mechanisms; or evolution. In my view these different types of analysis can be viewed as hierarchically ordered – and that answers to the more biological types of 'why' for any particular emotion will often help in answering the other types. (As an example, a possible evolutionary/functional answer to 'why do we cry?' is given in Section 11.2.)

It could be argued that, in concentrating on biology, we are throwing the baby out with the bath water; that we are in the position of the physicist whose explanation of the occurrence of a rainbow does not touch on the fact that it is beautiful. There are certainly those who would say that a rat cannot possibly have feelings like those of a human being and that to study the former will not enlighten us about the latter. This is a semantic red herring. The rat is not identical to the human. It may in some respects be totally unlike the human. But where there are similarities these may explain human behaviour to us, without forcing us to the conclusion that rats are small furry people. The detection of such similarities and the discovery of the extent to which they are meaningful can result only from our investigating the possibility as opposed to ignoring it. Where changes in the emotional behaviour of a rat (Wynne & Solomon, 1955) are paralleled by changes in self-report of emotions in people (Hohman, 1966) it can suggest a similar organisation of behavioural control (Chapter 11). Equally, where there are differences between species, appropriate (e.g. ecological) analysis of the differences can illuminate the reasons for the idiosyncratic behaviour of each.

It could also be argued that the study of animals cannot provide us with the kind of data which are provided by introspection – and introspection provides our best *a priori* reasons for treating emotion as an important topic. However, self-report, and presumably therefore introspection, often fails to reveal the true underlying causes of human behaviour (Schachter, 1980). The rat may therefore give us a clearer picture of humanity than does humankind especially if we are not distracted by the question of asking whether animals have emotions 'exactly like' those of humans.

1.3. Darwin and 'the expression of the emotions in animals and man'

Darwin in his studies of emotion preferred to observe animals rather than humans for this very reason – that they are 'less likely to deceive us'. He is often touted as the father of modern biology. Certainly, modern biology has a strong evolutionary flavour. However, in advocating a comparative approach, Darwin has an even better claim to being the father of the modern psychology of emotion. His book *The Expression of the Emotions in Man and Animals* (reprinted in facsimile, 1965) not only presents a good case for the genetic basis of emotional behaviour but also presents a variety of observations and opinions which can be seen as forerunners of contemporary research on emotion.

The bulk of his work analyses facial and bodily expressions. The important point for him was in each case to determine whether an expression was largely innate or largely the result of experience. Darwin suggested that 'whenever the same movements of the features or body express the same emotions in several distinct races of man, we may infer with much probability, that such expressions are innate'. He therefore posted a questionnaire to various parts of the world soliciting descriptions of expressions and the contexts in which they were produced to provide the data for such an analysis. He was of course mindful of the unifying effects of culture and, for example, specifically excluded a comparison of American negroes with Europeans on the grounds that their expressions might be similar for cultural rather than genetic reasons. Similarly, he studied the expressions of young children on the grounds that they would have had little time to learn complex expressions.

In this way he provided an essentially positive answer to the question of whether at least some expressions are common to particular emotion-provoking situations throughout the world. A corollary of this was his finding that the emotions portrayed in photographs of emotional expressions could often be accurately identified. Both for humans and animals, Darwin believed that this communicative aspect of emotional expressions was a major force shaping their evolution.

It should be noted that the expression of the emotions extended, for Darwin, well beyond facial expression, simple bodily attitude, or 'instinctive tendency to performance of an action' (op. cit., p. 30). For example, he pointed out that in 'almost all animals ... terror causes the body to tremble. The skin becomes pale, sweat breaks out, and the hair bristles. ... [Urine and faeces] are involuntarily voided ... the breathing is hurried, the heart beats quickly, wildly and violently' (op. cit., p.77). Thus, for Darwin, emotion generally resulted in quite widespread skeletal and systemic changes.

A strong genetic control of complex components of emotion of the type discerned by Darwin implies an extensive evolutionary history. This brings us to an apparent paradox in the analysis of emotion: the contrast which is often drawn between emotional and rational behaviour. If emotion is irrational, in the sense of counterproductive, why has it not been eliminated by selection pressure? The answer to this lies in the functional value which can be discerned in virtually all emotional reactions under at least some conditions.

1.4.   Cannon and the 'utility of the bodily changes in pain and great emotions'

Cannon is most frequently cited in the literature on emotion for his attack on James's theory of emotion (Section 1.5). However, an equally important contribution to an understanding of emotions is his analysis of the function of the physiological changes which accompany many emotional states. Peripheral autonomic and hormonal responses in emotion are often discussed largely in terms of their psychological consequences. Such discussion can result in the impression that peripheral reactions are present simply to confuse the psychologist, or to provide employment for psychophysiologists. However, as Cannon (1936) pointed out, such peripheral reactions are of great importance in readying particular organ systems for particular types of action and in returning such systems to a basal state when such readiness is no longer required.

Cannon itemises the 'increased blood sugar as a source of muscular energy ... increased (adrenaline) in the blood as an antidote to the effects of fatigue ... the vascular changes produced by the sympathico-adrenal system favourable to supreme muscular exertion ... the value of increased number of red blood corpuscles ... the changes in respiratory function (as) favourable to great effort ... the utility of rapid coagulation in preventing loss of blood' (op. cit., p. xiv).

Cannon's discussion of these issues centres on the physiological advantages of the bodily changes observed. The changes he considers can all be viewed as placing the animal into a state of readiness for events which are likely to accompany or follow particular emotional states.

For example, in many cases a situation which results in an animal becoming fearful is very likely to be one in which the alternatives are to run away or to get damaged, e.g. bitten. The release of adrenaline, according to Cannon would not only ready muscles for flight but also speed coagulation of blood released by a bite, hence reducing blood loss.

It could be argued that most if not all of the physiological changes which accompany emotion have such physiological utility. Certainly, some of the changes (in e.g. red blood corpuscles) discussed by Cannon are not ones of which psychologists normally take great account. What appears to a psychologist, then, as a particularly mysterious aspect of emotion may be so because it fulfils a largely physiological rather than psychological function. However, some psychologists have viewed physiological changes as more than epiphenomena of emotion.

1.5.   James and feelings as the basis for emotion

Darwin (cited in Mandler, 1984, p. 47) viewed internal physiological changes as necessary, integral parts of an emotional state – without such changes you would not have true emotion.

However, his approach seems to have been that some external stimulus, or a specific interpretation of an external stimulus, gives rise to a state of the central nervous system (the emotion) which then can have linked to it (by selection pressure) directed, communicative and internal responses. The emotion, on this view, precedes the responses both in evolutionary and functional terms. The opposite suggestion was made by James (1884) and phrased in a provocative way implying that bodily change necessarily precedes the occurrence of emotion proper (see Chapters 5 and 6).

There are two points worth noting about James's original statement of his position which can be lost sight of when considering the attacks on it. First, James was not talking about all emotions but only 'those which have a distinct bodily expression'. If we start from a Darwinian analysis of the evolution of complex behavioural patterns, we have every reason to suppose that some emotions could occur with little bodily change – since such change would not serve any function in the situations for which the emotion had evolved. Secondly, even for those emotions which have distinct bodily expression, James says 'without the bodily states following on the perception ... we might see the bear, and judge it best to run, ... but we could not actually *feel* afraid.' Normally, if we say that someone *is* afraid of the bear we imply both that they *feel* afraid and also that they will *act* afraid. James's theory purports to be about the feeling components of emotion in specific contrast to directed skeletal responses, and possibly also communicative expressions.

Viewed like this James could merely be making the trivial proposal that bodily changes result in feelings. His subsequent statement that these feelings *are* the emotion would then be a tautology based on a particular (fairly unusual) linguistic definition of emotion. The tone of James's writing implies a stronger position than this – and subsequent attacks on James have usually been addressed to the position that aspects of emotion such as expression are dependent on feelings. It is this view which Cannon (1927) specifically rejects since 'total separation of the viscera from the central nervous system does not alter emotional behaviour .. organic changes could not occur soon enough to be the occasion for the appearance of affective states' and a number of other similar reasons (Cannon, 1927; Chapter 5).

It can be seen that, to some extent, it is a matter of purely verbal definition whether, like James, we wish to say that feeling is essential to emotion. If we do so, we will then need some other word for states which are otherwise similar to emotion, so defined, but which are not accompanied by feelings. However, it is clear that however one chooses to define emotion, Cannon's arguments place severe constraints on the relationships which are postulated between feelings and emotions. These constraints could even be sufficient to persuade us to modify our definition of the word if the chosen definition forced us into cumbersome circumlocutions when discussing scientific facts. This is quite a likely occurrence since Cannon has drawn on data from a laboratory situation which is unlikely to be matched under normal circumstances and for which, therefore, colloquial usage may be inadequate. Laboratory research is not the only source of data which forces us to depart from our usual use of language.

1.6. Development of the emotions

Cannon's criticisms of the strong form of James's theory were based on data from adult animals – with the assumption that the control of emotion is essentially the same at all ages. Darwin, of course, specifically studied children because he assumed that adult responses were contaminated by changes which occurred during development. Research on the development of the emotions suggests that this is to some extent the case and that the historical order of appearance of the theories of James and Cannon may be matched by changes in the control of emotions during development. For example, one of Cannon's criticisms of James's position mentioned above was that the reaction of the viscera is relatively slow in comparison to the relatively quick responses people make to emotion-provoking stimuli. In young children however such responses are not quick. A child after banging its head against a table will pause for a few seconds, usually with no expression on its face and only after such a pause will start to cry. As most parents can attest, despite the long delay the resultant distress can none the less be very great. This type of delayed response can be seen for a surprising number of years.

Observations such as this suggest a complicated sequence in the development of the emotions. Initially, stimuli elicit visceral reactions with some delay, then 'frequent perception of visceral response leads to its symbolic representation. This means ... that after we have had much and varied experience ... we can think about this kind of stimulation, about the internal upset that represents this kind of emotional experience, and we can do it with rather short latencies' (Mandler, 1962, p.327). So, it can be suggested that James's analysis is basically right in young children and that the more complicated adult picture results from superimposition on this early type of response of additional behavioural control dependent on learning or maturation (see e.g. Mandler, 1984, p.234; Lyons, 1980).

1.7.   Learning and emotion

The importance of learning for emotion was fully recognised by Darwin. 'When there exists an inherited or instinctive tendency to the performance of an action, or an inherited taste for certain kinds of food, some degree of habit in the individual is often or generally requisite ... . The power of association is admitted by everyone [and] it is ... important for our purposes fully to recognise that actions readily become associated with other actions and with various states of mind.' In fact a large part of Darwin's endeavour was to try and distinguish those components of emotion which were innate from those which were learned. Likewise it is implicit in James's account that we learn which objects are appropriate as elicitors of particular emotions.

However, behaviour analysts, where they have been brought to think about emotion at all, have usually seen it as a side issue to the study of behavioural plasticity. Emotion pops up as a 'hereditary pattern-reaction involving profound changes of the bodily mechanism as a whole, but particularly of the visceral and glandular systems' (Watson, 1929, cited by Strongman, 1978, p.19) – inconvenient for the experimenter but not strictly relevant to the study of learning. The basic innate pattern reactions were in Watson's view 'certainly not the complicated kinds of emotional reactions we see later on in life but ... *form the nucleus out of which all future emotions arise*' (Watson, 1924, p.124, his emphasis). He also thought that the introspectionist bias which colours James's account of feelings 'gave the psychology of the emotions a setback from which it has only recently begun to recover' (op. cit., p.108).

Yet, for years behaviourist theories of learning have used motivational concepts which are highly relevant to the study of emotion – and these concepts may even have emotion words as descriptors. Radical behaviourists have done their best to avoid the use of concepts such as emotion but this does not make their data or their disguised view of emotion less relevant. More recently, writers in the behaviourist tradition have started to talk about emotion quite openly (e.g. Millenson & Leslie, 1979; Gray, 1971a; 1975) and I will argue later in this book that emotional as well as purely motivational factors are important in the learning of new responses.

The current view that the study of animal learning provides us with an analysis of the cognitive processes of animals (Dickinson, 1980) is also fruitful in two separate ways. The first is that it provides a method of objectively approaching and labelling the types of complex process which are usually termed emotional. The second is that in providing a means of relating animal cognition (i.e. the ways that animals relate items of information to one another) to human, it can bridge one of the major gaps in the comparative study of the emotions.

1.8   Cognition and emotion

The cognitive contribution to emotion has been emphasised by a number of authors recently (e.g. Mandler, 1975, 1984) – often starting with the idea that while the presence or absence of feelings may determine whether an emotion is felt, cognitive appraisal or evaluation will determine the nature of the emotion (Schachter & Singer, 1962; Lyons, 1980). Cognitive appraisal is clearly important in determining whether environmental stimuli give rise to an emotion, which emotion results, and what behaviour actually results from the emotion. For example, the capacity of a PhD *viva voce* examination to induce anxiety (see Section 11.8) clearly depends on cognitive evaluative factors. Likewise, even when an emotional state is produced in a reliable and reproducible manner by brain stimulation, the observed behaviour of the animal can depend markedly on its assessment of, for example, the status of other animals close to it (Chapter 2). However, the specific cognitive factors operating to determine the reaction of a specific individual to a complex environmental situation are beyond the biological limits of this book. The role of cognition in emotion, as opposed to the detailed mechanisms which give rise to particular cognitions, is considered in Chapter 5.

1.9.   Biology and emotion

Whatever is meant by the emotions, it is clear from our review so far that emotions are usually accompanied by skeletal muscular reactions and internal physiological changes the basic organisation of which are determined to a considerable extent by genetic factors. In many respects both emotional expressions and internal changes can be seen as being 'released' by stimuli. Innate releasing mechanisms, as studied by ethologists, are often seen as fixed motor programs which only require the specific releasing stimulus to trigger a stereotyped response sequence. Release of emotional expressions and physiological reactions might appear to set them apart from the directed skeletal responses, which also accompany emotion, but which in many cases are not as automatic as 'release' would imply. The next chapter investigates the concept of release in relation to emotion with a view to showing that quite flexible control of behaviour can be implied by the term – and concluding that a similar type of control can be assumed to operate for each of internal physiological response, communicative expression and directed skeletal responses.

The view that each of these types of reaction consists of motor or other programs which can be released by an appropriate stimulus or internal state is important when the evolution of emotion is considered. If the components of emotion consist of separable 'released' responses it is clear that they could have evolved initially in response to some basic, e.g. physiological, selection pressure. Once evolved for one reason, however, it is clear that they could evolve further in response to the presence in the animal's repertoire of those other reactions which often accompanied them. In the early stages of such evolution there is no reason to suppose that there would be any degree of integration of the control of the different components – indeed release of one type of component could depend on completely different stimuli from another. Subsequently, more integrated control could evolve where it was of advantage.

Consider emotional expressions. It seems clear that these are integrated aspects of emotional output which perform a straightforward communicative function. However, an evolutionary approach to expressions poses the question of how they could have evolved and why they currently take the form they do. Evolution by natural selection implies a gradual development of any evolved feature of an animal's form or of its behaviour patterns. In the case of communicative expressions both the capacity to send information in one animal and the capacity to receive and correctly interpret information in a second animal must evolve together. It will be argued in Chapter 4 that what are now communicative expressions may have evolved initially to ready the animal for classes of action which were frequently required when it found itself in a specific situation. Subsequently, some components of such expressions evolved further in response to social and communicative pressures, not directly related to the original selection pressure which gave rise to them – with in some cases a loss of the original function for which the expression was selected initially.

The genesis of the innate physiological changes which accompany emotion is clearer. For example, it was noted above that many of these fulfil the primary physiological function of placing organ systems in readiness for vigorous action. Each of the many changes could have evolved separately in response to the pressure to make the animal more efficient in agonistic situations. What is unclear in this case is whether such changes simply accompany emotions or whether they

play a significant part in the control of emotions or emotional behaviour. It is clearly possible that the controlling mechanisms of basic
physiological changes, and the changes themselves, could be involved
in further evolution; and could become critical components of systems
designed to place the animal in a state of mental or behavioural
readiness for vigorous action. The release of adrenaline, for example,
could be used to change the normal control of behaviour in the same
way that it changes normal cardiovascular control or changes clotting
of the blood. Likewise, inasmuch as its own bodily changes are perceptible to an animal, they could contribute to what we term emotional
feeling. They could then be subject to further evolutionary pressure,
depending on the consequences of this perception. Chapter 6 considers the question of how far physiological changes (and feelings if these
are not merely the result of such changes) simply accompany emotion
and how far they are integrated into the control of emotion. It is clearly
possible that even in humans the role of physiological changes in
emotion is under active evolutionary selection.

If this general view of the various changes which accompany, or
form part of, emotion is true, it makes it very probable that early on in
evolution the various components of emotion were under independent
control from each other. Given the different types of reaction we have
been considering (expressive gestures, physiological change and of
course coordinated responses like running away) and the potential
modifiability of these reactions by maturation and learning, it is clear
that we have no guarantee that, at the level of biological processes,
emotion will be a unitary construct, even in highly evolved organisms
including man. For example, given the complexity of natural stimuli
(such as lions) it is possible that under normal circumstances (i.e. those
commonly met with during phylogeny) certain internal and external
emotional reactions will occur together in a functionally fortuitous
manner – each reaction being triggered by a separate aspect of the
stimulus complex with no direct causal basis for their simultaneity.
Until we discovered their exact mechanisms, such reactions would
appear to be consequences of a single central state. After their
mechanisms were known they would have to be treated as functionally
separate.

While creating this problem, a specifically evolutionary approach
can also help to solve it. If we see a specific emotion as being a set of
reactions released by changes in some single central underlying control
system we may well be in error. If, however, we see a specific emotion
as being a set of reactions which have evolved to satisfy some common

purpose or goal, we have a means of approaching them which does not prejudge the issue.

Both 'released reactions' and 'purpose' as used in the previous paragraph need clarification. In the case of 'released reactions' we need to be clear about what kinds of elements of behavioural control could be subject to selection pressure. In the next chapter I will discuss the concept of release and its extension to 'state-dependent reflexes'. This provides at least some ground rules for considering the control of basic elements of emotional reactions. In Chapter 3, I will discuss the concept of purpose in the context of evolution, and since the connotations of words such as purpose and goal can be contentious, I will suggest the substitution for them of the more obscure but less loaded term, 'teleonomy'.

2: Releasers and state-dependent reflexes

The physiologists who, during the past few years, have been so industriously exploring the functions of the brain, have limited their attempts at explanation to its cognitive and volitional performances. Dividing the brain into sensorial and motor centres, they have found their division to be exactly paralleled by the analysis made by empirical psychology, of the perceptive and volitional parts of the mind into their simplest elements. But the *aesthetic* sphere of the mind, its longings, its pleasures and pains, and its emotions, have been so ignored in all these researches that one is tempted to suppose that if (physiological psychologists) were asked for a theory in brain-terms of the latter mental facts they might ... reply either that they had as yet bestowed no thought upon the subject, or that they had found it so difficult to make distinct hypotheses that the matter lay for them among the problems of the future, only to be taken up after the simpler ones of the present should have been definitely resolved.

And yet it is even now certain that of two things concerning the emotions one must be true. Either separate and special centres affected to them alone are their brain-seat, or else they correspond to processes occurring in the motor and sensory centres, already assigned, or in others like them, not yet mapped out.

William James: What is an emotion? (1884)

2.1. Apologia

The present chapter deals with basic concepts rather than details of specific emotional phenomena. As such it has a large neuroscience content. In this it contrasts with the rest of this book. Both the paucity of neuroscience in the work as a whole and the highly selected data in the present chapter require some justification.

2.2. Neuroscience and emotion – a brief digression

At the time I started to write this chapter exactly a century had passed since James published the views quoted at the head of it. Since that time the physiological psychologists have not ceased to 'industriously explore', and the sheer volume of potentially useful data from physiology and the neurosciences is enormous. Certainly, neuroscience has been crucial in helping our understanding of perception and motor control. However, a search for mechanism cannot easily proceed until the phenomena to be explained have been unambiguously categorised. In this sense physiology holds a mirror up to psychology. It provides a touchstone against which the more fundamental principles of a psychological theory can be tested. But it is no substitute for such a theory. Even in the area of perception purely psychological analysis has to define the explicandum (i.e. perception itself) before physiological analysis of feature detectors and so on can be related to object recognition. Even now, theories of the final stages of object perception depend heavily on psychology and cybernetics as opposed to physiology – although the physiological nature of the systems involved places extensive constraints on the details of such theories (see Frisby, 1979).

In Chapter 1 it was concluded that 'emotion' has not been clearly defined. This is particularly true at the relatively microscopic level required before a bottom-up physiological investigation can proceed. Of course, many texts, particularly in neurology, devote space to 'the limbic system and emotion'. However, in equally many cases this appears to have occurred because the definition of the limbic system has been as sloppy as that of emotion. The alternative, particularly in physiological psychology, is that emotion has not been treated generally. Rather, a chapter is headed 'the physiology of emotion' and then specific limited classes of behaviour are considered. When this has happened the emotions are usually itemised as sex, aggression and sleep! These are specific enough, and relatively easily defined. Unfortunately, not only is this list somewhat restricted, but, particularly with aggression, we have no reason to suppose *a priori* that what has been studied is an emotion as opposed to the consequence of a variety of emotions.

The bulk of this book, therefore, employs data from the neurosciences only where they seem pertinent to a particular argument.

2.3.   Neurophysiology and emotion

Electrical stimulation of the brain can produce fragmented chunks of behaviour, complex behavioural responses, and frequently what appear to be full blown emotional reactions. It is tempting, therefore, to see such stimulation as a simple way of dissecting out components of emotion.

Panksepp (1982), for example, sees electrical stimulation of the brain as a key to the emotions

based on the assumption that (electrically elicited) 'stimulus-bound' behaviours reflect species-typical expressions of class-typical brain circuits which mediate emotions, and, hence, that a realistic and scientifically useful taxonomy of emotions, in humans as well as other mammals, could be based upon the number of distinct behavioural control systems that can be activated in this manner. (op. cit.)

His object is to provide an economical description of emotion systems.

He first restricts his analysis to cases where stimulation produces skeletal, visceral and hormonal changes – together with changes in sensory receptive fields. He then notes that 'from a relatively diffuse zone centred around the dorsolateral hypothalamus of the rat, we can evoke feeding, drinking, gnawing, hoarding, predatory aggression and copulation'. We will consider in detail below evidence that stimulation at a single site can elicit a variety of behaviours depending on the animal's environmental situation – suggesting that a single central state can be responsible for the occurrence of a variety of behavioural reactions. Using an analogous argument Panksepp proposes that all of those different classes of behaviour which are elicited from the dorso-lateral hypothalamus are dependent on a single emotional state ('expectancy'), diffusely represented in the hypothalamus. He uses similar arguments to identify three other primary emotions: fear, rage and panic.

There are a number of points where this particular use of data from electrical stimulation of the brain appears unsatisfactory. The first is its isolation from other data. It may be that only four separate neural systems can be discovered in the hypothalamus (but see below). If this is so then it argues against such systems being central to the control of emotion. For example, Panksepp does not separate the control of feeding from that of copulation. Yet they are clearly separate in terms of external adequate stimuli, internal predisposing state, associated species typical behaviour patterns and virtually every other character-istic one can think of, other than the positive effect they have when used as instrumental reinforcers. While it may be that the hypothala-mus contains 'a unified executive sensory–motor system for the media-tion of exploration-approach-investigation' (Panksepp, 1982, p.415) this system must be one which can be activated by a variety of different emotions rather than being one in which activity constitutes the emo-tion. The supposedly magical effects of electrical stimulation have apparently blinded Panksepp to other sources of information.

A second problem is the assumption that an apparent lack of speci-ficity of the effects of stimulation in the rat necessarily implies uni-formity of the brain circuitry involved in the emotion related to the different elicited behaviours. First, stimulation could be having an effect akin to an increase in arousal, which simply increased the probability of observing behavioural output from a wide range of systems, the control circuits of which could be totally distinct. Second-ly, stimulation could well be simultaneously activating functionally discrete systems, the anatomical separation of which was not great. The apparent lack of specificity described by Panksepp in the small brain of the rat contrasts, here, with the specificity found by Flynn (see below) in the much larger cat brain, where totally different behavioural effects could be obtained with changes in electrode placement of as little as 0.5 mm. The possibility that, in the rat, a relatively large electrode is stimulating a variety of neurally separate structures simultaneously cannot be ruled out. A third problem is that in many cases the data Panksepp cites were obtained in studies which did not vary the animal's environment to determine the optimal eliciting stimuli for any particular reaction or which did not analyse the degree to which the optimal stimulus interacted with the electrode site in determining what reaction would be seen. He ignores this point and, while he cheerfully acknowledges the fact that quite discrete circuitry is involved in the control of quiet biting attack and other forms of attack (see below), he none the less says that it and other 'forms of predatory aggression are considered to be expressions of the foraging-expectancy system'. This is despite the fact that many forms of the cat's attack on a rat are not related to hunger in any way.

It is clear, then, that while electrical stimulation of the brain can provide us with useful information about the control of emotion its effects need to be interpreted with care. Its true value can only be assessed when the data are integrated with other sources of information. It may be of interest to note that while attempting to use electrical stimulation of the brain as a privileged source of information about emotion, Panksepp advocates the use of introspection as well as a second privileged source. A similar point can be made about both techniques. Each appears to offer an especially easy route to the understanding of emotion, but each is in reality a source of data no better, but possibly no worse, than any other. It is only by integrating the data across different research areas that we will be able to approach emotion in a coherent fashion.

In the remainder of this chapter, therefore, the neurophysiological data have been chosen to illuminate specific basic concepts in the study of emotion, those of 'releaser' and 'state-dependent reflex' rather than to attempt to solve all of the problems of emotion at a stroke. Likewise, the neurophysiological data will be presented in the context of an initial behavioural analysis.

2.4. Releasers and emotion

Before one can quantify behaviour, it is necessary to identify specific units or patterns of motor output. What is acknowledged as a specific behaviour pattern will be to some extent a function of the observer. But, particularly in phylogenetically simpler organisms, some behavioural reactions are so stereotyped that they have been termed fixed action patterns (see Hinde, 1966, Ch. 3). Stimulus control can often appear similarly simple. Action patterns of both a more- or less-fixed type are often reliably elicited by specific stimuli in the environment: the female tick drops on to the mammals on which she will lay her eggs in response to the smell of butyric acid; herring gull chicks beg for food in response to certain specific features of their parent's bill; and male sticklebacks will attack each other in response to their red bellies (see Hinde, 1966, pp.43–8). When such stimuli result in fixed action patterns they have been called releasers.

The terms fixed action pattern and releaser are convenient as a starting point for our discussion, but should not be interpreted too rigidly, especially in the context of vertebrate behaviour. The female tick may be reacting to an essentially simple stimulus, but the herring gull and stickleback react on the basis of a number of stimulus characteristics such as size, shape, colour and movement. The term releaser is justifiable in this context since the characteristics are a very limited subset of those available in the natural stimulus object, but initiation and strength of the behavioural patterns elicited depends on additive, and sometimes more complex interactions, between different stimulus characteristics. Likewise, fixed action patterns are not immune to some variation (the stickleback's behaviour will depend on that of its opponent, for example), and many variable behavioural patterns stand in the same relation to releasing stimuli as do fixed action patterns (see Hinde, 1982, pp.43–6).

In what follows, therefore, I will discuss release in a fairly general way. Classically viewed innate releasing mechanisms (sign stimulus – fixed action pattern) represent an archetype or idealised form of release for what follows but this should not imply that a division is to be, or can ever be, made between specific and general stimulus objects or between automatic and flexible responses. Further, the concept of release is particularly useful in the analysis of emotion if we add an additional source of variability – central reaction. We can view a specific emotion (or component state contributing to it) as the releaser, with the eliciting environmental stimuli at one remove from this.

In the previous chapter we discussed communicative emotional expressions, systemic changes, and directed skeletal responses. It is my contention that, in many instances, reactions of all these types should be viewed as released, or enabled, by specific emotional states.

In the case of communicative emotional expressions, their identification rests on a degree of stereotypy of response and it is also reasonable (see Chapter 4) to see specific expressions as being tied to specific emotional states or stimulus situations. It is less obvious that physiological responses in emotion are either stereotyped or that specific patterns of physiological response relate to specific emotions (Chapter 5). That physiological reactions can be both stereotyped and fairly tightly stimulus bound, however, can be shown even in humans.

For example, the let-down reflex occurs in response to contact by an infant with its mother's nipple. Sensory nerves register the contact and send a signal to the mother's brain. This results in the release of the hormone oxytocin which, in turn, when it reaches the nipple through the blood stream, allows milk to be released. Stimulus control is quite specific in that physical contact with the nipple other than by the infant does not generally produce the response. 'For human mothers this reflex response to suckling frequently becomes conditioned to baby cries , so milk appears promptly at the start of nursing' (Rosenzweig & Leiman, 1982, p.192). Given the presence of this endocrine reflex and its conditionability, it is not unreasonable to suppose that other hormonal and physiological systems could be under equivalent control and hence contribute to emotion. An obvious exocrine example is salivation which can occur not only in response to the presence of food in the mouth but also to stimuli such as odours associated with food and even to mental imagery of food items in the absence of external stimuli directly associated with food.

Finally, while skeletal behaviour (e.g. a flight reaction in response to a fearful situation) could be viewed as being released by an emotion, it is clearly much more complex than a fixed action pattern, even if this term is extended to cover, for example, the stickleback's behaviour. It appears, therefore, to be the least describable in terms of release of the various concomitants of emotion. This problem will be dealt with in the rest of this chapter.

2.5.   Reflexes and goal-directedness

The terms release, unconditioned reflex, conditioned reflex, fixed action pattern and the like all carry an implication of rigidity of behavioural sequences. The borrowing by psychologists of the word reflex has been particularly unfortunate in this regard. As colloquially used, e.g. of the knee jerk, it implies automatism. Yet the stretch reflex, which is the basis of the knee jerk, is actually a feedback system designed to maintain the current position of the limb in the face of varying external circumstances. With more complex behaviour the idea of a reflex, while still technically correct, appears to have forced psychologists into an excessively mechanistic as opposed to cybernetic view of behavioural control.

The preface to a recent volume on the neurophysiology of motor coordination makes the following points:

The lone overnight flight of a ruby-throated hummingbird across the Gulf of Mexico is a migratory behaviour mediated through an incredibly lengthy, repetitive series of wing movements, each movement being produced by a complex sequence of muscle contractions. It is significant that these same movements may be used to mediate other behaviours, and that these same muscle contractions, in different sequence, may be used to produce other movements … . A laboratory rat may learn to perform an escape behaviour in a shuttle box, bringing its performance to a high level of efficiency by modifying its movement on successive trials. After intraperitoneal injection of pentobarbital sodium in an amount sufficient to render the animal severely incoordinated, the escape behaviour is still performed, albeit through a different sequence of movements, even to "rolling" out of the compartment in response to the warning signal. The lesson is that, even though the topography of the movements making up a behaviour may be much the same each time the behaviour occurs, the animal is not restricted to that particular sequence of movements in carrying out the behaviour.

(Towe & Luschei, 1981)

Many units of behaviour, from the simple reflex to highly complicated systems, can be described in terms of the following basic model: some condition is tested; a departure from the desired value causes action which is repeated until the condition is satisfied; finally, achievement of the desired value allows control to pass to some other system (Hinde, 1966). The application of this model requires care, particularly with simple systems, since termination of a behavioural sequence may be due simply to the fact that it has previously occurred rather than being due to termination of feedback error signals (see Hinde, 1966, Chapter 3). Where the model is applicable, however, behaviour can be described as being in some sense goal directed. 'If rats are subjected to spinal or cerebellar operations so as to interfere with their motor coordination, they may nevertheless use quite novel movements to make errorless runs through a maze … the new movements are not stereotyped, but selected from variable patterns in such a manner as to bring the animal nearer the goal' (op.cit.).

The running of the rat in the maze, described above, is usually termed a conditioned instrumental response. Yet the effects of the lesions described by Hinde, and much other evidence (e.g. Dickinson,

1980), suggest that it is not the response sequence *per se* which is conditioned but rather the tendency to seek the goal.

At a more detailed neuronal level, the analysis of such organs as the cerebellum has led to the view that

the generation of motor movements must arise in the CNS from a set of components of an intended movement vector, probably assembled by many structures of the brain at a particular time... The intended movement vector must be placed in the context of the functional state of the body at a given moment. Such 'putting into context' requires that this vector interact with ... the *status quo* of the motor system, such that the intended movements be adequate to achieve the desired goal ... . The way of achieving the same goal may be different, depending on the initial posture, as in writing a letter on the blackboard when one's arm is immediately in front, and in writing a letter when one's arm is almost totally stretched out. The sets of muscles utilised under these two conditions are different; however, the letters are very much the same, indicating that the *intended movement* is the same whereas the mechanism of execution is rather different.

(Llinas & Simpson, 1981, my emphasis).

It should be noted that the 'intended movement vector' can be viewed simply as a motor command, but specified within the same coordinate system as is used by sensory feedback. Although much more complex than the stretch reflex, it is similar to it in that it implies that motor output can be adjusted by feedback from changes in environmental circumstances to achieve or maintain some specified end state of the system.

2.6.   Electrical stimulation of the brain and goal-directed behaviour

It is in this context that we will discuss the physiological analysis of the release of directed behaviour. The starting point for this work is the now classical observation that removal of the cortex can result in displays of what is usually referred to as 'sham rage'. The affected animal growls and spits. The hair on the back of its neck will rise and internally it shows all the bodily signs of rage. However, the rage is unusual in that the animal is not faced with the environmental stimuli which would elicit rage in a normal member of the same species and also the rage does not appear to be directed at any specific environmental target. The observation of sham rage implies that actions which we would normally call aggressive are generated subcortically, although directed cortically. Flynn (1967) describes a series of experiments designed to analyse the subcortical neural basis of aggression in cats through the application of electrical stimulation. A critical feature of Flynn's approach, in comparison to some others, is insistence on analysing the eliciting properties of electrical stimulation as opposed to its reinforcing properties. A corollary of this is his manipulation of environmental stimuli so that the state created by the electrical stimulation has available to it a variety of objects which could be adequate stimuli for the release of the behaviour.

Cats differ in their tendency to attack and kill rats. Some can be placed in an enclosed area with a rat for a long time without the rat coming to any harm. Others will attack the rat – and when they do so the form of attack is characteristic of hunting rather than of the attack the same cat might make on another cat. The approach to the rat is usually called quiet biting attack. In Flynn's typical experiment a cat, chosen for not attacking rats spontaneously, would be placed in a cage with a rat. Stimulation of medial portions of the hypothalamus and the midbrain causes the cat to attack the rat in the quiet biting manner. 'The response is comparable to a reflex in its regularity, although it is by no means as stereotyped as most reflexes. The directed nature of the attack is clear, because a stimulated cat will chase a rat around the cage, and jump at it if the rat is clinging to the wall' (Flynn, 1967). More lateral electrode placements also produced attacks on the rat but rather than being 'quiet biting' attack, stimulation at these sites elicited vocal and other signs of rage and was aversive. However, it did not necessarily result in severe damage to the rat. Stimulation of yet other sites can give rise to an attack not on the rat, but on the experimenter (Flynn, 1969), so that the direction and nature of attack can be determined within a particular cat by suitable choice of electrode.

With sites that elicit quiet biting attack the cats have preferences for specific targets. Anaesthetised or stuffed rats will support attack to a much greater extent than other objects of a similar size. Among such other objects the cats are more likely to attack a hairy toy dog than a styrofoam block. In the absence of stimulation the animal does not attack any object. Even with stimulation the cat will only make an attack if certain objects are present and the extent to which it will attack appears to depend on how closely an object approximates to the usual adequate stimulus for such attack in the wild. We have then what can be described as a 'state-dependent reflex' (Note 2.1). Stimulation of the medial hypothalamus creates a state in the presence of which a reflexive behavioural sequence can occur. To borrow from computer terminology we could say that the state 'enables' behaviours. Which particular one of a set of enabled behavioural sequences is observed in any particular situation depends on the extent to which adequate stimuli are present and, in the case of a stimulus such as a rat, on the behaviour of the stimulus.

We need not, however, view this behaviour as goal directed in the highest sense. Cats have a highly developed sense of smell, and yet placing a blindfold on them produces a large reduction in the number of attacks they will make on the rat. On the other hand removing their sense of smell has no such effect. Thus, the electrical stimulation appears not to issue a command of the form 'attack any rat you can detect', but has an effect which is in some way modality specific. One possibility, suggested by additional experiments from Flynn's laboratory, is that the stimulation affects sensory processing – perhaps making supernormal stimuli which already have a subthreshold capacity to elicit attack.

Flynn (1967) found that touching certain areas of the muzzle during electrical stimulation of the medial hypothalamus elicited head movements to bring the object into contact with the lips, and that touching the lips elicited jaw opening. The critical finding for our purposes was that the size of the area from which such responses could be elicited increased with the intensity of hypothalamic stimulation. By analogy, the effects of the stimulation on the visually guided components of attack could have occurred also through enlargement of the receptive field for the adequate visual stimulus.

Flynn, himself, concludes that his stimulation is activating a 'patterning mechanism'. This mechanism produces a variety of effects.

First is a direct effect that accounts for motor responses ... that appear to be relatively independent of environmental conditions: examples are walking, sniffing, snarling, and the display of rage. Second is a motor disposition. If an adequate stimulus is present a second response ... appears. Examples are attack on a rat and the effect of hypothalamic stimulation on jaw closure. If one stimulates the motor nucleus for jaw closure and obtains a response of a given size, the response will be found to increase with concurrent stimulation of the site in the hypothalamus from which attack can be elicited. Stimulation of the hypothalamus facilitates jaw closure at the level of the motor nucleus.

(Flynn, 1967)

The importance of discriminating between behavioural sequences unconditionally elicited by electrical stimulation and those conditionally elicited depending on the presence or absence of adequate stimuli is also shown in experiments by Delgado & Mir (1969). Using radio-controlled stimulators, they tested monkeys which were free in the home colony with other monkeys or were in operant testing apparatus. They emphasise that certain isolated aspects of emotional behaviour can be elicited by brain stimulation separated from the total pattern normally associated with emotional reactions. An example of this was an 'aggressive expression induced by stimulation of the brain stem between the facial and trigeminal nuclei. The effect could not be conditioned, was not accompanied by offensive–defensive behaviour, had no positive or negative reinforcing properties, and did not modify social behaviour in free monkeys. This effect contrasted with the appearance of well coordinated and purposeful aggressive responses evoked by stimulation of other tectal and thalamic structures' Delgado & Mir (1969). In this case, therefore, we have stimulation releasing an isolated element of an aggressive display which we, and indeed the other monkeys, can deduce is in no way due to aggressive intent.

By contrast, Delgado & Mir's observation of the effects of stimulation-induced attack parallel Flynn's in showing the necessity for the presence of an adequate stimulus – but in a more subtle form. They found that whether or not stimulation elicited threat and attack behaviour depended on the social ranking of the monkey concerned. The structure of the colony was manipulated by removing dominant animals and replacing them with submissive ones. When the stimulated animal was lowest ranking stimulation induced negligible amounts of agonistic behaviour by her, but did result in a considerable amount of agonistic behaviour being directed towards her. As her social rank improved stimulation produced increasing amounts of agonistic behaviour in her, largely directed towards lower ranking individuals. Thus, the state induced by stimulation enabled a set of reflexes one of which was triggered not so much by another monkey, in general, but by a monkey which could easily be beaten up, in particular.

The results obtained by Flynn and by Delgado & Mir, taken together, show that the elements of emotional behaviour are likely to be organised in an essentially hierarchical fashion. Specific components of expression (e.g. facial) can be released by stimulation in an unconditional fashion – and, when they are, they generally occur in isolation from other components which would normally accompany them. Directed sequences of behaviour can also result from stimulation, but these sequences are not generally released by the stimulation itself. Instead, the stimulation enables sets of reflexes, different ones of which can then be released depending on the presence of different adequate environmental stimuli. Adequateness of a stimulus in this context reflects (in the monkey at least) the *interpretation* put on a stimulus by the organism rather than any crude aspect of its simple physical configuration. As suggested above it seems useful to think of these directed patterns of behaviour as state-dependent reflexes. It should be emphasised that in many cases state-dependent reflexes and indeed other reflexes, must be viewed as relatively plastic, goal-directed activities (I believe that Flynn remarks somewhere that not only does the experimenter perceive a cat attacking a rat to have a goal, the rat acts as though it shares this view!). How far an *emotion* can be viewed as a state capable of enabling reflexes is a question to which we will return in later chapters.

2.7.   Electrical excitation versus natural excitability

We have seen that variations in the effects of stimulation within an individual depend on the supply of adequate environmental stimuli. We also need to take into account variations between individuals in the extent to which electrical stimulation is necessary to induce the behaviour in the presence of a constant adequate environmental stimulus. Flynn, for example, specifically chose for his experiments cats which did not spontaneously attack rats. In later work Flynn delineated both a system within the brain which elicited attack behaviour (e.g. Chi & Flynn, 1967) and also a second system which could inhibit attack, and which appeared to be involved in defensive behaviour. A question arises from these various findings. 'Can one explain the observation that not all adult domestic cats spontaneously attack and kill formidable self-defensive prey (rats) by the fact that cats differ in the extent to which they are intimidated by rats? ... . Furthermore, if such variation exists, can it be related to the excitability of the attack suppressive system revealed by Flynn?' (Adamec & Stark-Adamec, 1983).

Adamec & coworkers have carried out a variety of behavioural and neurophysiological studies which show that cats do vary along an aggressive–defensive personality dimension of a fairly general type (determining responses not only to rats but also humans, novel environment, and other cats). This dimension was found to relate to responsiveness of cells in the amygdala and, most importantly, this personality characteristic of the cat could be changed by modifying the excitability of the amygdala and related circuits.

2.8.   The neural basis for the release of behaviour

It is common in the ethological literature to refer to sequences of behaviour as being released. However, it might seem that it would be better, when discussing the effects of electrical stimulation of the brain, to refer to elicitation. I have kept to the use of 'release' for two reasons. First, it retains the idea that the behavioural sequences observed are in some sense submerged within the animal and are allowed to surface when appropriate prior conditions are met. Secondly, it seems likely that they are in fact released – that is to say that under normal circumstances the occurrence of such behavioural sequences is actively inhibited by higher centres and the behaviour occurs as a result of removal of this inhibition. 'Release' may usefully refer, then, not only to the effects of some external adequate stimulus but also to other ways in which the inhibition of a motor sequence can be removed.

A classical example of such removal occurs during the copulation of the praying mantis. The male mantis is smaller than the female and both are insectivorous. It turns out, therefore, that after the male has initiated copulation the female starts to eat him from the head down. The result of 'losing his head' is instructive. The head contains circuits which inhibit the fixed action patterns of mating, while the circuits which contain the blueprint for this behaviour are located lower down. Thus, copulation continues not so much in spite of, but because of, the loss of the head (see Gould, 1982). We can view the copulatory motor program, then, as permanently ready to take over the mantis's musculature but continually held in check from on high.

The occurrence of sham rage (Section 2.6) is an essentially similar mammalian example. It is most easily accounted for by presuming that rage is normally inhibited by cortical circuits and that the removal of the cortex results in a general release of aggressive behaviour.

Roberts (1984a) has proposed that most behaviour is controlled in this way.

The point of view taken is that the nervous system is highly restrained, with inhibitory neurons acting like reins that serve to keep the neuronal 'horses' from running away. It is proposed that in coherent behavioural sequences, innate or learned, preprogrammed circuits are released to function at varying rates and in various combinations. This is accomplished largely by the disinhibition of pacemaker neurons whose activities are under the dual tonic inhibitory controls of local circuit and ... projection neurons coming from neural command centres.

(op.cit.)

There is considerable evidence in favour of such an arrangement of neurons (see Roberts, 1984a,b and papers cited), which need not concern us here. An important detail of Roberts's model for our present purposes is that it 'requires that decrease or cessation of inhibitory signals ... would be a necessary, but not always sufficient, condition for the firing of (command neurons). The latter might begin to fire spontaneously when partially or completely relieved of inhibition ... or excitatory input ... might be required. In the latter instance, less excitatory input would be required ... in the absence of inhibition ... than in its presence' (op.cit.; see Figure 2.1). Even with the simplest neural circuits, therefore, we have the possibility that a particular stimulus can both produce simple release of behaviour and also, at

Tonic suppression   Adequate stimuli

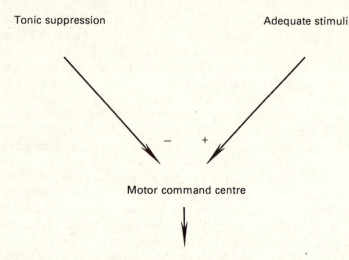

Motor command centre

Organised output

Figure 2.1. Roberts's model of the control of motor output. A motor program which will result in organised motor output depends on a command neuron. Under normal circumstances the command neuron is held in check by tonic suppression. A reduction in suppression need not result in activation (release) of the motor program but could instead enable specific adequate stimuli to activate the program. However, an intrinsically active command neuron could initiate the motor program in the absence of adequate stimuli. Variations in the intrinsic properties of the command neuron (e.g. in response to hormones) could shift the effects of removal of tonic suppression between releasing and enabling. Similarly, 'supernormal' stimuli could well initiate the program even with normal levels of tonic suppression of the command neuron.

some other time, enable release by some additional stimulus. Which effect would be produced would depend simply on the extent to which the enabled command neuron was spontaneously active. It is particularly noteworthy that the same input could both unconditionally release one circuit and enable a second circuit. A corollary of this is that we need not expect release and enabling to be logically distinct. The same state could well enable a state-dependent reflex on one occasion, and unconditionally release essentially the same motor program on a second occasion when the command neuron had become intrinsically more active and no longer needed input from a specific adequate stimulus. This view could encompass both the effects of varying levels of deprivation on the types of stimulus which can elicit certain behaviours and also such phenomena as displacement activities.

This point is particularly relevant given the role of hormones in emotional behaviour.

Acetylcholine, the catecholamines, serotonin, neuroactive peptides, prostaglandins, and steroids in many instances may serve to optimise regional nervous system activity in relation to functional demands without themselves being involved in specific information transmittal. They exert chemical actions that influence the efficacy of the information-transmitting functions in the mainline and command circuits. Some peptide or steroid hormones, for example, may temporarily 'line-label' neural pathways, differentially facilitating behavioral options related to consummatory activities such as eating, drinking, and sex.

(Roberts, 1984*b*)

Thus, the extent to which particular groups of behaviours are released by environmental stimuli (via, say, incentive motivation) and the extent to which they are released by changes in internal state could depend on changes in sensitivity or spontaneous activity within a single neural command circuit. Separate neural circuits for internally and externally controlled behaviours would not be required.

2.9.   Releasers, state-dependent reflexes and emotion

The effects of electrical stimulation of the brain reviewed above suggest that simple, relatively stereotyped sequences of output from particular effector systems are preprogrammed and can be released by stimulating appropriate critical points of the nervous system. In the case of expressive behaviour it is clear that these sequences represent fragments of the behaviours which would occur normally. More complex, goal-directed, patterns of output – involving the integrated activity of several effector systems – can be obtained by stimulating other points in the brain. These state-dependent reflexes depend on available environmental stimuli for their release and for the exact form of their execution. What is released, therefore, appears to be an intended movement vector (in the sense used by Llinas & Simpson, see Section 2.5) or some higher order equivalent.

This does not imply any specific organisation of the emotions. Nor (Section 2.3) does it imply any special status for electrical stimulation as a source of information about emotion. We have no evidence to compel the view that the electrically generated state which enables a state-dependent reflex has to be equated with an emotional state. Nor is there a clear dichotomy between the state-dependent reflex and the simple unconditionally elicited behavioural sequence which might be presumed to be a component of such a reflex – some electrically generated sequences of behaviour are simply more plastic than others.

However, releasers and those states which generate complicated state-dependent reflexes can be seen as units which could be subject to evolutionary pressure. In the context of emotion, autonomic reactions, hormonal reactions, facial and bodily expressions, and directed skeletal responses could all depend on equivalent organisation and be subject to independent selection pressures. Given a goal-oriented command structure, it is also likely that an integration of such different types of response could be selected for. We should be prepared, therefore, for:

1. Independent control systems, which appear to act in concert simply because they have evolved in the context of a particular environmental situation.
2. Integrated control systems, which do in fact act in concert because of a common central control structure.
3. Partially integrated control systems, which may be in the process of evolving from independence to integration. It is particularly important, given the tendency of humans to view themselves as the pinnacle of creation rather than merely one more evolved species, that we should be prepared for this third possibility in the control of human emotions.

Given the uncertainty as to the degree of integration of the systems which are involved in emotion, we return to the problem mentioned in the first chapter of how we might organise the data until such time as we can resolve the question of whether, at the process level, an emotion is a unitary, identifiable condition or state of the organism. It was suggested that, as a working device, emotions could be viewed as groups of reactions which can be related to a common teleonomy (evolutionary purpose). Exactly what is meant by this is the subject of the next chapter. But it should be emphasised that the 'goal' of a particular reaction as it has been discussed in the present chapter has no direct relation to the 'purpose' of the same reaction as discussed in the next. Where the goal of a rat is copulation with a member of the opposite sex the evolutionary purpose will be transmission of genes to the next generation. The rat may well pursue its goal with fervour even when the evolutionary purpose is prevented by, for example, sterility. Thus, in the present chapter we have been discussing intended movement vectors – specific neural activity which effectively codes a motor program in terms of the feedback signals which will terminate the program (much as appropriate feedback terminates changes in output from the stretch reflex). In the next chapter we will be discussing the evolutionary pressures which have resulted in the instantiation within the nervous system of particular intended movement vectors and the like.

3:   Purpose and emotion

There lived a happy coelocanth
In dim primordial seas,
He ate and mated, hunted, slept
Completely at his ease.
Dame Nature urged: 'Evolve!'
He said: 'Excuse me Ma'am,
You get on making Darwin,
I'm staying as I am'.

Horace Shipp: The coelocanth

3.1.   Teleonomy, a redefinition of purpose

In the previous chapter we discussed the release of behaviour patterns
in terms of general control mechanisms without considering how and
why such mechanisms might have evolved. In his preface to the 1965
edition of Darwin's book Lorenz cites as a key to modern behavioural
biology 'the fact ... that behaviour patterns are just as conservatively
and reliably characters of species as are the forms ... of bodily structures; ... (they) unite the members ... of taxonomic units ... (and) can
become "vestigial" or "rudimentary" just as the latter can. Or on
losing one function they may develop another.'

The idea of purpose has for many years been problematic in biology.
However, it is possible to discuss some classes of purpose in biology
from a scientific point of view – by referring to 'purposes' which
specifically exclude the existence of any purposive entity as their
source. One such alternative is 'function' as used by Lorenz.

Functional explanations do one thing that no mechanistic explanation can:
They can explain similar outcomes produced by different means. For example,
the eyes of vertebrates and octopi are very similar in many ways: Both have
lenses, a retina, and some means of limiting the amount of light that can enter.
This convergence cannot be explained by common ancestry or any similarity of
developmental mechanisms. The *only* explanation we can offer for this asto-
nishing similarity is the common function of these organs as optical image-
formers. Because convergence is such a common phenomenon in evolutionary
biology, it is no wonder that functional explanations are so common and so
powerful there.   (Staddon, 1983, p.7)

Monod (1974) presents the same argument more controversially:

It would be ... arbitrary and pointless ... to deny that the natural organ, the eye, represents the materialisation of a 'purpose' – that of picking up images – while this is indisputably also the origin of the camera. It would be all the more absurd to deny it since, in the last analysis, the purpose which 'explains' the camera can only be the same as the one to which the eye owes its structure. Every artefact is a product made by a living being through which it expresses, in a particularly conspicuous manner, one of the fundamental characteristics common to all living beings without exception: that of being *objects endowed with a purpose or project*, which at the same time they show in their structure and execute through their performances (such as, for instance, the making of artefacts).

Rather than reject this idea (as certain biologists have tried to do) it must be recognised as essential to the very definition of living beings. We shall maintain that the latter are distinct from all other structures or systems present in the universe by this characteristic property, which we shall call *teleonomy*... .

By the autonomous and spontaneous character of the morphogenetic processes that build the macroscopic structure of living beings, the latter are entirely distinct from artefacts, as they are, moreover, from the majority of natural objects.

(Monod, 1974, pp.20–2, his emphasis)

Taken in this light, purpose or teleonomy is simply a descriptive property of a system. It is distinguished from other properties normally ascribed to systems, biological or otherwise, by being in part historical and in part projective. Instead of being a property which relates directly to the system as it is now, teleonomy implies a potential endpoint for the system. This endpoint is that which the effective goals (in the form of intended movement vectors, etc, see previous chapter) built into the animal's control mechanisms are likely to achieve, subject to the natural world remaining within certain limits. Unfortunately, the word purpose is for most people indivisible from the idea of an agent of the purpose. Further, to talk of purpose in relation to animal behaviour could be to imply that the animal itself is the purposer. Neither of these implications is true of teleonomy in Monod's sense (it has been said that an organism is a gene's way of fulfilling its purpose of making more genes). In an attempt to leave behind the idea of a purposive agent I will, therefore, use the more esoteric term teleonomy; since it seems to me useful to explore the implications of viewing emotional systems from a teleonomic perspective.

3.2   Teleonomy versus teleology

Before proceeding we should first distinguish teleonomic explanations from teleological ones. Teleological explanations have had a checkered career in philosophy, as is shown by the extensive arguments and counterarguments in a recent collection of papers which starts with the definition that 'teleological explanation is that form of explanation that uses some future state to explain some current state' (George & Johnson, 1985, p.ix). It is certainly not usual to explain the present in terms of what will happen in the future. Teleonomic explanations, however, are explanations in terms of function and as such refer to future states in only a restricted manner.

Functional explanations can, in principle, be reduced to mechanistic ones: Given perfect understanding of the principles of genetics and development and complete information about evolutionary history, we can, in principle, reconstruct the process by which the shark achieved its efficient form. For this reason the biologist Pittendrigh (1958) suggested the label *teleonomic* (as opposed to *teleological*) for such accounts. ... In practice of course, the necessary detailed information about mechanisms is often lacking so that we must settle for functional accounts and hope that they are teleonomic ones.

(Staddon, 1983, p.6, his emphasis)

As Staddon emphasises, functional/teleonomic explanations, while incomplete in themselves, will often lead to mechanistic explanations. It is my contention that this is the 'function' that they themselves can fulfil in the study of emotion.

It is important, therefore, that in describing systems in terms of teleonomy we should not allow everyday implications about purpose to clutter our arguments. Equally importantly, teleonomy should not be invoked in a casual way whenever the scientist thinks he perceives a glimmer of sense behind one of Nature's more wonderful contortions. Rather, our ascription of any particular teleonomic property to a system should be based on objective data and analysis. One type of such data, as shown in Staddon's discussion of the function of eyes, is comparative. This is particularly important for psychological investigations because it can be carried out on extant organisms. Another sort of data is the fossil record. Here the psychologist is at a disadvantage since behaviour does not readily fossilise. (But see, for example, Leakey, 1981 for a discussion of the deduction of some behavioural characteristics from patterns of wear on teeth and similar items.) However, where a physical structure has evolved for, say, a display function some clues as to the course of the evolution of the behaviour may be provided by fossils. A final potential source of information is in the sequencing of genes which has started to provide us with estimates of the genetic relationships between different species. If, in the future, the relationships between genes and innate behavioural control mechanisms are discovered, then gene sequencing could provide a critical source of information.

For both molecular systems which have the capacity to express

themselves as living beings, and motor systems which have the capacity
to express themselves as motor acts, it has proved fruitful to use
projective concepts of a similar type to teleonomy. As was emphasised
above, such concepts do not provide causal explanations. The complete causal explanation of, for example, the migratory flight of the
humming bird or the rolling of the intoxicated rat (Chapter 2) will be
immensely complicated. The advantage of purposive explanations of
such behaviour is that they are concise and easy to handle. What would
be the consequences of viewing emotions as teleonomic systems?

3.3.   Emotions and teleonomy

First, we should note that the mechanisms of heredity, and hence the
effects of mutation and selection, are essentially conservative. An
entire organ system or behavioural control system is unlikely to appear
out of the blue. Rather, mutations make gradually available in a new
context structures which already fulfil some function in an older context. We should be prepared, therefore, for a certain degree of overlap
in the control systems involved in different emotions. This will most
obviously be the case when two separate emotion systems share some
common requirement. For example, if both need the body to be
prepared for vigorous activity, we would expect a partial, if not total,
overlap in the autonomic and hormonal reactions involved. At the
same time, we should not be surprised if some released reaction, which
is of utility in relation to one emotion, is also released by some other
emotion and thereby subserves a somewhat different function (Note
3.1).

Secondly, we should be prepared for variation in the extent to which
skeletal, autonomic, hormonal and expressive effector systems are
necessarily involved in any particular emotion. Although it is not
common usage, there may be considerable heuristic value in treating
as emotions all those complex states of the organism which involve in
their functioning predominantly innate reactions of any two or more of
these effector systems. We need not presume that all emotions, nor
any particular emotion at all times, need involve all of the effector
systems. This idea could well necessitate further departures from the
usual use of the word emotion. Thus, it may prove useful to consider
moods as emotions (they are usually distinguished from emotions by
being more long-term and less discretely elicited): for example, depression in adults could well depend on the inappropriate release of a
system present in the young animal to conserve energy when it is

separated from its care giver (Kaufman & Rosenblum, 1969). Likewise, some apparently simple reactions such as the let-down reflex in human mothers (Section 2.4) may be associated with sufficient motivational, cognitive and skeletal responses that we would wish to see them as being released as part of, as yet, un-nameable emotions.

Thirdly, we should be prepared for some independence in the control of different components of specific emotions. The release of hormonal and skeletal responses, for example, could have evolved independently, but in such a way that under virtually all circumstances normally experienced by an animal in its natural environment they would interact cooperatively. In the laboratory, then, appropriate manipulations could separate functionally components of what one would wish to continue calling, from a teleonomic point of view, a single emotion. This situation may well be exemplified by Hofer's experiments, described in Chapter 8, on the heart rate and behavioural responses elicited by removal of the mother.

Fourthly, it should be clear that a teleonomic view of emotional systems does not preclude an important role for experience in their development, nor does it preclude an interaction of emotions with conditioning. The reverse is the case. Although innate patterns can provide a solid foundation for the development of structures (physical and behavioural), the capacity for adaptation to variable environmental conditions is clearly of advantage. Two physiological examples which underscore this point are: 1) the extent to which hardness of the skin of the hands depends on the use to which we put them; and 2) the adaptation of our thermoregulation to higher or lower ambient temperature via, among other things, changes in our metabolism.

Fifthly, in relation to all of the foregoing it should be emphasised that the teleonomic value of an act or of a bodily change can in no way be equated with the purpose for the act given by self report (see especially Schachter, 1980) or by any specific use to which the act, or bodily change, is currently put. The foregoing might suggest that each emotional system should be studied in isolation as each is likely to be idiosyncratic in its teleonomy. However, in practice external constraints on the evolution of such systems appear to have generated many common features in their overall 'design'. There is, therefore, likely to be considerable value in comparing emotions within species. This is especially true if the control systems for different emotions share access to smaller scale releasing systems of various kinds. Particularly at the neurophysiological level, the detailed working out of some behavioural sequence in relation to one emotion may transfer directly to a second emotion once it is determined that the same intended movement vector (Llinas & Simpson, 1981) or higher order command is issued by both.

All of the above are suggestions as to what we might expect to find using research techniques which are current in the study of emotion. At the technical level, emphasis on teleonomy would suggest that more reliance should be placed on comparative (phylogenetic) investigation than has been usual – except perhaps in the study of facial expression. (An example of both the changes in perspective which can be produced by such an approach, and of the technical problems involved in it, is given by a tentative analysis of why we cry in Section 11.2.)

3.4.   Teleonomy and its implication for a unitary view of emotion

In one sense a teleonomic view of emotion can integrate what might otherwise be thought of as separate systems. Thus, for each specific class of effector system (e.g. skeletal, autonomic, hormonal) an emotion could be viewed as a state of the organism. The parallel organisation of the control systems of these different classes, coupled with the orderly arrangement of the environment, would mean that a particular state of one effector system (say the autonomic) would normally be accompanied by a particular state of other effector systems except in very unusual circumstances. From this point of view, an emotion would be a set of such coincident organismic states, different emotions being distinguished on the basis of different teleonomies. However, teleonomy and parsimony, taken together, strongly imply that until we can prove otherwise we should be prepared for emotions to reflect single states which have common control over all the relevant effector systems. The parsimony of a single state view of emotion is clear. From the point of view of teleonomy, it seems to me that a single system with an unitary goal is likely to be more efficient than a committee of subsystems, each with its own independent goal, whose action adds up under normal circumstances to an implicit common goal. At the moment we have virtually no data to allow us to choose between these views. However, one reason for taking the multiple system point of view seriously is the variety of divergent views of emotion to be found, each reflecting some specific area of research. Rather than assume that researchers in different areas are studying identical underlying processes, it is necessary for us to demonstrate experimentally either their identity or else the relation between them. The advantage of teleonomic analysis is that it allows us to discuss the various effector systems in relation to emotion without prejudging whether the cooperativity that we normally see between such systems is the result of some single central nervous control centre, or is the result of separate control centres (which natural selection, coupled with consistencies in the external environment, causes to act in concert under normal, but not necessarily abnormal, environmental conditions). A teleonomic view of these systems leads directly to the question of which of these alternatives is in fact the case in any specific instance.

Providing an answer to this question would require researchers to work simultaneously in what have previously been separated areas. In the remainder of this book we will discuss the present state of such areas and attempt to interrelate them. Before proceeding, a final disclaimer should be made about the value of teleonomic argument. Determining teleonomy with any degree of certainty is extremely difficult. Teleonomic considerations do not provide us, therefore, with a solution to the problems of emotion. Rather, consideration of teleonomy gives us a framework within which to phrase questions and, as in the case of the points made in Section 3.3, can lead us to expect more complex kinds, or different kinds, of relationship between control variables than we would normally consider. Teleonomic arguments, accurate or inaccurate, will give us a new perspective on what *might* be the case; but types of analysis other than teleonomic are required to determine what *is* the case in any specific instance.

4: Expression: a window on the emotions?

Your face, my thane, is as a book where men

May read strange matters. To beguile the time,

Look like the time; bear welcome in your eye,

Your hand, your tongue: look like the innocent flower,

But be the serpent under't.

William Shakespeare: Macbeth

4.1. Why do emotions produce expressions?

Common experience suggests that emotional states are reflected in facial and bodily expressions, and that in some cases specific states may result in specific, identifiable, expressions. It would be parsimonious if we could assume that an emotion releases a facial expression (Chapter 2). However, unlike organised skeletal responses or internal physiological change, facial expression has neither a direct physical effect on the external environment nor any obvious function with respect to the internal environment. The main function of expressions can be presumed to be communication (see Chevalier-Skolnikoff, 1973, p.20). Particularly with human beings, therefore, it is possible that expressions would be deliberate rather than reflexive and that the form of an expression could be easily learned rather than being innate (cf. the different gestures used in the various sign languages). How closely particular expressions are linked to particular emotions, the extent to which they are learned, and the extent to which they do in fact convey information, are all important questions.

The fact that expressions are largely there to be seen makes noting down when they occur fairly straightforward – particularly if we are not initially concerned with whether a specific expression is emotional or not. However, any change in an animal's situation as a result purely of its expressions will depend on the interpretation of those expressions by other animals. This makes teleonomic analysis of an expression more difficult.

This analysis is greatly aided by judicious interspecific comparisons and such comparisons have been made widely. As Darwin put it: 'the view that man had been created with certain muscles specially adapted for the expression of his feelings struck me as unsatisfactory. It seemed probable that the habit of expressing our feelings by certain movements, though now rendered innate, had been in some manner gradually acquired' (Darwin, 1965, p.19). In considering interspecific similarities of expression we should bear in mind what is known about similarities of physical form. Similar structures (whether parts of the body or parts of the behavioural repertoire) occur in different species for at least two different reasons. First, the species may be genetically related – in which case the similarity of structure need not be matched by similarity of function. (For example, humans have an appendix as the vestigial remains of the caecum of our early forebears, not because our digestion requires its presence.) Secondly, convergent evolution, may have taken place, the nature of the structure being determined by its required function – in which case the similarity may tell us about that overall function but may not reflect similar microstructure. (For example, bats and birds are both adapted to flight by modifications of the forelimb and can be contrasted with flying squirrels who use a different method. However, bats and birds are essentially phylogenetically unrelated having 'discovered' flight independently. The detailed form of the adapted limb differs markedly.) We need always to be on the look out, then, for structures which are the result of adaptation to a new function (flying) of some precursor which may have evolved for a different function (walking/grasping). Expressions are particularly subject to this process since any characteristic bodily movement which evolved for some functional purpose can inadvertently act as a form of communication. The effects of such communication will then enter into the adaptive equation both for the sender and for the receiver. The importance of signal value in evolution can be seen in the ridiculous plumage 'chosen' by many birds to attract their mates.

Darwin enunciated a number of general principles which he thought guided the evolution of expressions. The first of these is the principle of serviceable associated habits: 'certain complex actions are of direct or indirect service under certain states of mind ... whenever the same state of mind is induced ... there is a tendency for the same movements to be performed, though they may not then be of the least use'. His examples of this include the cat which 'treads' to display pleasure (treading in kittens being a method of obtaining milk) and the lifting of a forepaw by many dogs when they are attending (a gesture which could be preparatory to cautious approach). His second principle is that of antithesis: 'when a directly opposite state of mind is induced, there is a strong and involuntary tendency to the performance of movements of a directly opposite nature'. Examples of this are the position of a dog's tail, or of many animals' ears, which are held up when the animal can be presumed to be in a positive emotional state and down when it is in a negative one. His third principle was that of direct action of the nervous system. 'Of course, every movement we make is determined by the constitution of the nervous system; but actions performed in obedience to the will, or through habit, or through the principle of antithesis are here excluded'.

This is rather a catch-all for actions which are not easy to explain on the basis of the previous two principles. The example given by Darwin is that of trembling as part of fear. It can be seen that this does not fit the principle of serviceable associated habits as it has no obvious utility. It does not fit the principle of antithesis since it is not the opposite of any obvious reaction in states antithetical to fear. It seems, therefore, best explained as a kind of side effect of fear reactions – a result of the constitution of the nervous system not explainable in terms of any particular teleonomy of its own.

Andrew (1965) provides an argument which illustrates selection for a communicative function. With many animals flattening of the ears against the head could reduce the chance of damage to them during a fight. We might presume that reflexive flattening of the ears could then result through natural selection. Andrew points out that 'ear flattening, originally only a reflex act of protection, becomes potentially a device of communication'. This communicative function can then be selected for in its own right. Thus, 'in higher primates ear flattening is less pronounced and less significant... . They retain as a significant signal, however, retraction of the scalp which is a part of the movement in primitive flattening of the ears. In macaques and baboons, scalp retraction is much exaggerated and produces a spectacular display ... these displays ... have no elements of physical protection; their sole function is communication' (Andrew, 1965; see also Andrew, 1963). As we will see below, arguments such as this have to be treated with some care. However, an immediate question for many people, even given the truth of the above argument, would be: how relevant is it for human expression? What reason have we to suppose that the complex facial expressions we use are genetically determined as opposed to simply learned?

4.2.   Are human expressions innate or acquired?

What we require to answer this question is a source of data from which the effects of learning can be excluded. One such source is the observation of individuals for whom learning of expressions is *a priori* unlikely.

First, we can consider children who are born both deaf and blind. One would think that they had little chance to pattern their behaviour through observation of others. Also, in most cases it is unlikely that complex expressions could have been trained in them by their care givers. Blind and deaf children, none the less, smile, laugh, weep, stamp their feet, clench their fists and frown like normal children. A second group of interest are the mentally retarded. 'Even severely mentally handicapped children smile, laugh and weep although it is impossible, even with great effort to teach them to eat with a spoon. It is unthinkable that they could have learned these complicated motor patterns, when failing in tasks that are much simpler' (Eibl-Eibesfeldt, 1971). Even relatively complicated sequences of expressive behaviour may be innate. 'That more is innate than is often supposed was demonstrated to me by a ten-year-old girl born blind, but with perfectly good hearing ... . I payed her a compliment. She immediately blushed and turned her face briefly towards me and then looked down, just as any sighted girl does when she feels bashful' (op. cit.). Such patterns even occur when one would presume that behavioural training would be directed towards its suppression. '(Blind) children also develop a whole range of "bad habits" – for example typical human angry behaviour. Certainly no one has taught them this nor can they have had the opportunity to feel adults who were stamping their feet, clenching their fists and looking angry' (op. cit.). A number of workers have made essentially the same observations in this area – the expressions used by blind children are similar in form to those of sighted children, although there can be differences in the intensity of those expressions (see Ekman, 1982, pp.68–9, 152).

A different kind of evidence, providing the same conclusion, is that from cross-cultural studies. Given the different habits and rearing techniques in different cultures one can argue that any constancy of expressions, and of interpretation of expressions, across cultures argues for their innateness; while, of course, variations are suggestive of a developmental origin.

Research on cross-cultural identification of expressions (see below) argues indirectly for constancy of expression. If expressions were not in fact consistent, cross-cultural identification of expressions would be very difficult. Less research has been carried out directly on the constancy as opposed to the identifiability of expressions. However, careful analyses have been carried out by Eibl-Eibesfeldt (1971) and Ekman and others (see Ekman, 1982, pp.137–41). Both based their analysis on moving photographic records.

Eibl-Eibesfeldt used a camera adapted to take pictures at right angles to the direction in which it appeared to be pointing. He thus obtained film of 'candid' personal interactions in a wide variety of cultures. He emphasises that 'what the person did before and after being filmed and in what social context the behaviour pattern in question took place' was carefully recorded to eliminate subjectivity in assessment of the interpretation of the context of the expression. He identified a variety of expressions and actions which occurred in the same social context in different cultures – and which were often highly stereotyped (see Plate in Eibl-Eibesfeldt, 1971).

Ekman's group used a laboratory rather than ethological approach. They compared Japanese and American subjects who were asked to watch a stress-inducing film and also a neutral film. Psychophysiological and self report data were used to check that some kind of emotional reaction had been obtained in the subjects. Expressions were assessed with the 'Facial Affect Scoring Technique' a system which separately assesses movements in different areas of the face (see below). It is not yet clear whether the emotion categories used by this system are definitively related to specific underlying emotional systems. However, 'even if the facial behaviour were mislabelled ... the question is whether the repertoire of these different types of facial behaviour, whatever the label, is similar when subjects from these two cultures are in the same eliciting circumstance'. The correspondence between Japanese and American expressions in this study was extensive.

We should not conclude that emotional expressions will always occur in a similar fashion to specific stimuli in different cultures. Ekman *et al.* took care to use an eliciting situation which was likely to generate the same emotion in their two groups – and we shall see in Chapter 9 that, even with rats, the nature of a stimulus is less important for the control of behaviour than the interpretation that experience may have put on it. Equally important for the control of expression are the display rules operating in a culture. The Japanese and Americans were interviewed about their reaction to the film by a member of their own culture. This was unlike the film viewing situation – in which they were unaware that their expressions were being studied. In the interview there were marked differences between the two groups, with the Japanese showing happier expressions. The results overall are consistent with the view that the form of emotional and other expressions is innate; that particular expressions will tend to accompany particular emotions in unconstrained circumstances; and that, as might be expected given their communicative function, the expression elicited by a situation can be deliberately modified to change the message.

More extensive observations have been made on the capacity of persons from one culture to judge the nature of the emotion expressed by a person from another culture (see Ekman, 1982, pp.147–52). A problem in this area (see below) is in obtaining 'pure' examples of the expression of particular emotions. When care has been taken to use photographs for which there is good agreement within a culture as to the expression portrayed, then cross-cultural identification has been good. This has been true even with studies of preliterate cultures which have no acquaintance with the mass media.

Only a small number (happiness, anger, disgust, sadness, fear/ surprise) of types of emotional expression have so far been conclusively identified in this way. However, it is not unreasonable to expect that more may be identified (e.g. Ekman & Friesen, 1986, provide data which suggest that 'contempt' should be added to the list and is distinct from disgust). For example, the use of moving rather than still photographs could well improve identification (see discussion of the Facial Action Coding System below). Similarly, care needs to be taken in separating out culturally general and culturally specific communication. To take a non-emotional example, while a downward head movement is used virtually universally to signify assent (perhaps as a modified submissive gesture), dissent can be signalled by either a sideways (e.g. America) or an upwards (e.g. Turkey) movement of the head. It is tempting to see the dissent gesture as being culturally generated as the opposite of a more innately determined assent gesture, with opposite being translated slightly differently in different cultures. However, if there was only one convenient opposite gesture available we might think, erroneously, that both were innate. For this reason, it is not entirely clear that an assenting nod is itself innate or whether it may be derived from some more general innate tendency.

While it is clear that greater differentiation of recognised emotions might be obtained, we should also bear in mind the possibility that cultural universality may only apply to expressions generated by a limited number of discrete emotions and that the variety of emotions normally reported could reflect varying contributions from these.

4.3.   The description of expressions

To describe an expression as a smile is to prejudge its nature. We should consider, therefore, how we can define separate expressions. The answer which I would favour is in terms of the muscle groups and patterns of movement of those muscles employed in any particular expression.

Darwin (1965) placed considerable emphasis on the analysis of the action of different muscle groups in assessing expression. In fact, expressions can be reproduced to a surprisingly large extent by electrical stimulation of a single appropriate muscle group. A reasonable facsimile of the smile, for example, can be produced by stimulation of the *zygomaticus* (op.cit. Plate III) – although Darwin is careful to point out that the normal smile involves several additional muscle groups. Later workers, by contrast, have tended to ignore the anatomy of the face and also the objective measurement of facial changes and they have concentrated more on the information which human observers have been able to deduce, often from still photographs. However, as noted above, expressions are likely to have evolved from functional gestures and vestigial components of such gestures may remain. It seems entirely possible, therefore, that there are components of facial (and of course bodily) activity which could be detected by careful analysis but which could in no way be perceived by the average human observer in a naturalistic situation. This possibility, the greater objectivity of the analysis of muscular action, and the greater ease with which such analysis can be transferred to non-human primates (see Chapter 11) all argue in favour of such muscular analysis.

Unfortunately, at the practical level, it is difficult to measure the activity of the facial muscles through techniques such as electromyography while maintaining a natural context for the person in whose expressions one is interested. This is especially true since expressions can vary depending on whether the subjects know that they are being monitored. A compromise solution to this problem can be obtained nonetheless. Thus, Ekman and coworkers (see Ekman & Friesen, 1982) have developed a measurement system, based on anatomical considerations, but using still and moving pictures as the input data. They term this the Facial Action Coding System (FACS). FACS has a number of clear limitations deriving from the nature of its input. It cannot measure muscle activity which does not produce a reasonable amount of facial movement. In some cases the action of two or even three separate muscles appeared so similar that they had to be grouped together as a single 'action unit'. Also, the reliability of scoring, while high, is not 100%. A further disadvantage is that it requires both training and considerable effort for execution. The main advantage of the system, even in its present partially developed form, is its objectivity. It is intended to score movements of the face quite independently of any hypotheses one might have as to why the movements occurred. Further, 'the muscular basis of appearance change ... helps to overcome the problems caused by physiognomic differences. Individuals differ in the size, shape, and location of their features and in the wrinkles, bulges or pouches that become permanent in midlife... . Emphasis on recognising movements helps to deal with variations caused by physiognomic differences' (op.cit.).

In relation to the use of movements in FACS's scoring it is worth noting that movement alone may provide considerable information about expression. Bassili (1979, cited by Krech, Crutchfield, Livson, Wilson & Parducci, 1982) placed white dots on faces and then obtained moving photographs such that only the dots but not the other facial features could be seen. From the movement of the dots alone the emotional expression being portrayed could be identified, and there was some suggestion that, in the case of surprise, movement was one of the critical factors in its ordinary identification.

Use of FACS shows that there are many distinctions which are lost in our ordinary descriptions of expression. Of particular interest is the fact that FACS distinguishes 180 distinct forms of human smile (Ekman & Friesen, 1978, cited by Redican, 1982). This clearly adds some uncertainty to estimates of homology of the smile with primate expressions such as the play face (see Chapter 11). Redican (1982) points out that in pursuing this problem we need not only to analyse human expressions carefully but also to carry out similar muscular coding of primate expressions. It is a surprising fact that ethologists, normally careful to maintain objectivity in their data, report expressions in only loosely descriptive terms and often label them in ways (e.g. smile, play face) which prejudge their function rather than describe their objective configuration in terms of specific patterns of movement of specific muscles.

4.4.   Identical forms of expression with different teleonomy

The need for descriptions of expressions which do not prejudge their teleonomy or apparent current function is most obvious when we consider the voluntary control of expressive gestures. It may well be in the interests of some social group that their members come equipped with a variety of standard communicative expressions. However, natural selection operates on individuals rather than groups. Note that, in addition to facial and bodily expression of emotion, there is good evidence that emotional vocalisation is to some extent genetically determined (Malatesta, 1981). We can all think of occasions, particularly with human vocalisation, when it is to the advantage of the individual, and hence to his genes, of suppressing communication or indulging in active deceit. This may outweigh the advantage to the group, which is only indirectly related to the genes of the individual, of unambiguous communication (Note 4.1). Although deceit has not been well studied in animals other than man, there are clear indications that it does occur (see Redican, 1982, pp.268–71); and everyone can think of human instances of deceitful expression.

Of particular interest in this context is the fact that deliberate and involuntary facial expressions depend, at least at the higher levels, on separate neural systems. Thus, human patients can present with lesions which entirely paralyse voluntary but not involuntary facial expressions, while others have the reverse problem (see Ekman & Oster, 1979, p.547). Similarly, voluntary and involuntary expressions appear to have a separate ontogenetic development presumably due to differing rates of maturation in components of these different systems, particularly in relation to the capacity to imitate expressions at will (Ekman, Roper & Hager, 1980). There is also evidence that voluntary, but not involuntary expressions are to some extent lateralised, affecting the left hand side of the face to a greater extent than the right (see Hager, 1982). If we see lateralisation as a sign of recent phylogenetic development, this neurological picture is consistent with the idea that the evolution of deceit was subsequent to the evolution of expression. It remains to be seen whether voluntary expressions are generated in a different way, at the motor program level, from involuntary ones. It would seem more economical, however, if voluntary and involuntary 'commands' could release the same basic motor programs, at least unilaterally.

4.5.   Is there a one-to-one link between an expression and an emotion?

The deliberate production of expressions is one clear case where we would want to suppose that the link between a facial expression and the equivalent emotion is rather tenuous. We should also bear in mind that there may be no direct link between a specific emotion and a specific expression. If, for example, the signal value of an expression relates to the probability of a specific class of behaviour, then that expression should be released by all emotions which can enable such behaviour. There could also be non-specificity of control of expressions despite the accuracy with which expressions are recognised. The accuracy of recognition could be accounted for if a particular emotion, A, released one component of expression in common with a second emotion, B; and tended to release some other component of expression in common with a third emotion, C. Thus the signal value of the combined expression components could be unique to A despite the fact that the control of the individual components was in no way specific to it.

In the same way that an individual expression need not be unique to a particular emotion, an individual emotion need not be associated with a single expression which varies only in intensity. While, at the level of underlying process, a specific emotion may tend to give rise to a specific expression, at the level of behavioural output this expression could become admixed with elements of the expression associated with some other emotion which was being simultaneously generated by the situation. There seems, indeed, good evidence that expressions of basically different sorts can combine to produce distinctive blends (see Figure 4.1, p.50).

The changes in expression in the figure are attributed by Chevalier-Skolnikoff (1973) to changes in the intensity of anger on the horizontal axis and to changes in fear on the vertical axis (Note 4.2). Whatever the labels applied, it seems clear that the generation of such expressions must be viewed as multi-dimensional. It follows that the description by an ethologist of an apparently distinct expression does not imply that the expression is necessarily the result of a distinct emotion different from emotions associated with other expressions.

Thus, despite the fact that the form of expressions has a strong innate component, expressions do not provide us with a foolproof way of differentiating between different emotions, nor are they so structured that we can tell which expressions if any are in fact emotional and which are not. This uncertainty of categorisation of the peripheral skeletal activity which results in expression is matched by equivalent uncertainty in relation to directed skeletal responses and also peripheral autonomic or hormonal activity. We turn to a detailed consideration of the latter in the next chapter.

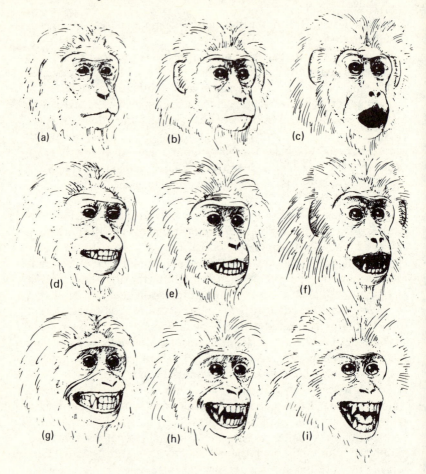

Figure 4.1. Expressions formed by blending of two basic types of expression. (a) Neutral; (b),(c) Increasing tendency to fight; (d),(g) Increasing tendency to flee; (e),(i) Increasing tendency to both fight and flee. Reproduced, with permission, from Chevalier-Skolnikoff (1973) 'Facial expression of emotion in nonhuman primates'. Original artwork by Eric Stoelting.

5: Are physiological changes epiphenomena of emotion?

There are many lies in the world, and not a few liars, but there are no liars like our bodies, except it be the sensations of our bodies

Rudyard Kipling: Kim

5.1. Why do physiological changes accompany emotion?

The work of Cannon discussed in Chapter 1 centred on pain and fear as 'great emotions'. It is also now obvious that 'in the natural state and particularly in subhuman species, the aggression, attachment and sexual patterns are usually accompanied by autonomic discharge … . The same functional stimuli activate the behaviour pattern and the autonomic nervous system arousal' (Mandler, 1975, p.136). Cannon suggested, essentially, that most such changes can be viewed as physiological preparations for the situation facing the animal. Even with the broader selection of emotions presented by Mandler, this view is unlikely to be contentious in either mechanistic or teleonomic terms.

Let us consider mechanism first. Particularly with examples like the let-down reflex or salivation (Section 2.4) to guide us we can accept that certain stimuli or the interpretation of those stimuli could result in activity in either the autonomic nervous system or glands under nervous control. The release of compounds such as adrenaline or direct action of the autonomic nervous system can then produce extensive changes in the animal's physiology which can involve increased muscular power, decreased bleeding, etc. The role of physiological changes in the gentler or subtler emotions may be more difficult to determine – but there is no reason at present to suppose that it will be markedly different.

Teleonomic argument here follows directly from mechanism. As Cannon argued, the physical changes which are the end product of the mechanism we have described improve the chances of the animal's survival in situations requiring great effort or which involve the risk of damage. Outflow from a particular branch of the autonomic nervous system, the release of a compound from a gland and similar events could be selected for independently; and, for example, once the release of adrenaline into the blood stream was occurring to trigger one particular physiological change, relatively minor changes in appropriate organ systems could allow selection in favour of control by adrenaline of additional reactions. So, while the physiological changes which we observe in the 'great emotions' are complex this complexity could clearly have resulted from the progressive accretion and modification of simple units.

Provided, therefore, that we are dealing with straightforward physiological end products we have no great problem with either the identification of the basic mechanisms of the physiological changes which accompany emotion or the construction of a reasonable teleonomic argument.

5.2. Could physiological changes play a role in emotion?

It seems very likely that at least part of emotional feeling is related to the physiological changes which accompany emotion. This is evidenced by such locutions as 'trembling with fear'. One obvious possibility, therefore, is that physiological changes occur for the teleonomic reasons given in the previous section, and that they happen to give rise serendipitously to feelings but that they have no further involvement in emotion than that.

However, I have already argued that once a compound such as adrenaline is acting as the trigger for one reaction it can easily become the trigger for others. We should not be surprised, then, if neural or hormonal reactions, or the physiological changes which result from them, became through further selection critical components of psychological responses. This would have two important implications. First, the psychological function of a particular physiological change could represent a phylogenetically later addition to a preexisting reaction. We should then expect a great overlap between the physiological changes which accompany emotions which are essentially different except that they have some common physiological requirements. Likewise, we should expect divergence of the physiological changes accompanying those same emotions in as much as their particular physiological requirements differ. It is also clearly possible that for some emotions the relationship between bodily changes, physiological function and psychological function could be different from the relationship for other emotions depending on their exact evolutionary history.

In this chapter I will consider the types of physiological response which accompany emotion and the significance of such changes for what are usually termed feelings. In the next chapter I will consider the question of the extent to which such physiological changes or feelings play a role in the generation of emotion and emotional behaviour.

5.3. Autonomic and hormonal discharge in emotion

The autonomic nervous system consists of two opposing subsystems – the sympathetic and the parasympathetic divisions. These innervate the pupils of the eyes, airways in the lungs, the heart, digestive system, bladder and genitals. In addition, the sympathetic, but not the parasympathetic, division innervates the adrenal medulla, liver, kidneys, spleen, muscles which constrict blood vessels, and muscles which produce piloerection. The parasympathetic, but not the sympathetic, division innervates the salivary and lacrimal glands (Figure 5.1). In general terms we can view the sympathetic division as placing the body in a special state of readiness and the parasympathic as returning the body to normal once the need for readiness has gone. It is common to think of autonomic discharge in terms of undifferentiated arousal, but a moment's consideration of the above list of target organs will show that this must be nonsense. There are differences between the two divisions in their specificity in that 'sympathetic reactions tend to be widespread affecting the responses of the organism as a whole, where-as parasympathetic reactions can be restricted to particular organs or glands' (Kandel & Schwartz, 1985, p.219). But even sympathetic reactions show some differentiation (see Section 5.7).

There is a huge amount of evidence for the involvement of the autonomic nervous system in emotion – none of it particularly clear as to psychological implications. While direct action of the autonomic nervous system on target organs such as the stomach or the intestines could clearly play a role in generating feelings, the prime target in this regard is likely to be the adrenal medulla. Activation of the sympathetic input to the adrenal medulla causes the release of adrenaline and noradrenaline into the bloodstream – with resultant widespread changes in the organism.

The situation is rendered more complex by the relatively specific release of non-adrenal hormones in situations in which the autonomic nervous system is also active. Other than adrenaline and noradrenaline which are to a large extent controlled by autonomic input to the adrenals, hormones have not received a lot of attention in the literature on human emotion. However, there is a large literature on the release of hormones in response to external stimuli and on their importance for subsequent behaviour in all species including man. These range from relatively simple reactions such as the let-down

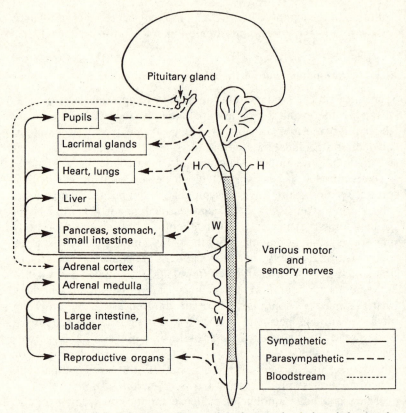

Figure 5.1. Cross-sectional view of the brain and spinal cord showing the outflow of the autonomic nervous system. This is divided into two parts: the sympathetic and the parasympathetic. They innervate most of the organ systems of the body with some variation in the target organs of each division. The sympathetic division derives from a middle portion of the spinal cord (shaded in the figure), while the parasympathetic division derives from the two ends. Thus the sympathetic division can be selectively transected as it was by Wynne & Solomon (1955; see W–W in figure). Surgical sympathechtomy leaves the sensory and motor nerves of the spinal cord intact. Transection of the spinal cord as occurs in paraplegic patients can also result in sympathetic denervation as in Hohman's (1966; see H–H in figure) study. In this case the parts of the body affected depend on the level of the lesion and there is a concomitant loss of sensory and motor innervation as well as sympathetic.

reflex discussed in Chapter 2; through more complex, but still relatively brief changes in, for example, the pituitary–adrenal system; to relatively long term hormonal changes which can affect and in turn be affected by interaction with other individuals and their hormonal reactions.

In what follows I will deal with autonomic and hormonal influences in parallel. But it is worth emphasising the separate nature of the systems despite their often concerted actions. Mason (1975) goes so far as to say that beside the skeletal and autonomic systems 'the endocrine apparatus ... represents a *third effector or motor system* of the brain'. Nor is this third effector system particularly simple. In discussing the complex interactions of hormones and behaviour it should particularly be borne in mind that the release of any hormone is likely to have widespread effects on other glands (see Leshner, 1977, for a concise discussion).

For the sake of simplicity, and to provide the greatest comparability with autonomic reactions, the following discussion is restricted to a single hormonal system – the pituitary–adrenal system. This system is directly related to the types of response with which Cannon was concerned. It also emphasises the parallels between autonomic and hormonal responses since the adrenals are a target of both autonomic and hormonal outflow.

The adrenals consist of two main parts: the medulla, which is activated by the autonomic nervous system to release adrenaline and the adrenal cortex which is a target for adrenocorticotropic hormone (ACTH) released from the anterior pituitary gland. ACTH causes the adrenals to release corticoid hormones (corticosterone in rats, cortisol in man) into the bloodstream. Adrenaline is the compound which has usually been exogenously administered in experiments which attempt to simulate the physiological changes which accompany natural emotions.

5.4. Emotional feeling after the elimination of peripheral feedback

It has often been assumed that neural feedback of bodily changes provides a major source of the feeling component of emotion. An obvious way to test this possibility is to eliminate such feedback by, e.g. spinal section (H–H in Figure 5.1). Unfortunately, given the paralysis which accompanies such an operation, it is difficult to test whether an animal's emotions, and especially its feelings, are affected by it. However, verbal reports from human beings are available.

Early reports suggested that emotional behaviour, inasmuch as it could be observed, was unchanged in patients with spinal transections. For example, Dana (1921) reports the case of a quadraplegic woman whom he saw 'showing emotions of grief, joy, displeasure and affection. There was no change in her personality or character'. However, he does suggest that while bodily sensations may not be essential for the expression of an emotion they 'extend and perhaps intensify the emotion'. The importance of peripheral feedback for reported feeling and for other aspects of emotion is emphasised in a much cited study by Hohman (1966; for other reports see Jasnos & Hakmiller, 1975; McKelligott, 1959, cited by Jasnos & Hakmiller, 1975). In discussion with others he had reached the tentative conclusion that paraplegics were generally unwilling to talk to intact persons about their reactions to the lesion, in case they were viewed as abnormal. However, Hohman, being himself a paraplegic, expected that he might get fuller cooperation than other investigators – and, indeed, some subjects who had previously been interviewed by a non-paraplegic experimenter gave different replies to Hohman on the grounds that he would understand their position better. (This demand elasticity of the responses shows how cautiously we must treat Hohman's own findings.) He found that

1. Individuals with spinal cord lesions report significant decreases in experienced emotional feelings associated with sexual excitement, anger, fear, and an overall estimate of emotional feeling, as compared to those experienced before injury.
2. Such subjects report a significant increase in emotional feelings related to sentimentality.
3. The data further indicate that, in spite of decreases in some emotional feelings, overt emotional behaviour may continue to be displayed.

(Hohman, 1966)

There was some indication that the reported lack of feeling could interact with the normal course of the other aspects of the emotional reaction, viz. 'I get kinda mad one minute, and the next minute it'll be like nothing happened. Seems like I get thinking mad, not shaking mad'. Further, it appeared that apparently normal expressive behaviour in these patients was the result of conscious attempts to manipulate people's reactions rather than the direct result of any internal change in state. 'I yell and cuss and raise hell, because if you don't do it sometimes I've learned people will take advantage of you, but it just doesn't have the heat it used to'. Hohman suggests that the normal emotional expression seen in sympathectomised animals is also due to 'acting'. In the light of the Wynne & Solomon experiment discussed in Section 6.2, it seems more likely that emotional expression, like other skeletal responses, is relatively independent of feeling except in as much as feeling may modify the intensity of any central eliciting state.

5.5.   Do visceral reactions differ in different emotions?

The above data suggest that peripheral physiological changes play a role in the generation of emotional feelings. James suggested a more specific hypothesis: that it is variations in the nature of bodily changes that determine our differing perceptions of different felt emotions.

Cannon's objection to this suggestion was that the same visceral changes occur in different emotional states – and that such changes can occur in states which are not emotional. Three points should be noted here.

1. Relatively minor quantitative variation in the relative balance between a few underlying physiological changes could easily give rise to a variety of quite distinct emotional sensations. The perception of colour provides us with an example of this type of phenomenon. The activation of only three colour channels is sufficient to result in many more than three distinct perceived colours and which colour is perceived depends on differences in the relative activity in the different channels.

2. The pattern of physiological changes in response to various stimuli can be highly consistent within an individual and yet vary extensively between individuals. Taking means across subjects in this situation could easily obscure differences in pattern which are highly discriminable to the subject (Schnore, 1959).

3. Failure to detect a differential pattern of peripheral change may be due to failure to measure the right variable. Many studies concentrate on sympathetic nervous responses, ignoring parasympathetic, and virtually none take measures which might reflect hormonal release.

We will consider first the evidence for the selective release of hormones (keeping to the example of the pituitary adrenal system) and then discuss, at greater length, the more contentious issue of whether specific patterns of autonomic discharge occur in relation to particular emotions.

5.6.   Emotion-specific release of hormones

That hormonal release can be both stimulus-specific and follow the type of time course associated with emotional reactions is shown by, for example, the let-down reflex. Whether in this case we would want to relate such release to emotion is a separate question. In other cases of hormonal release a hormone can maintain a high level for a long period of time (weeks or months), as does the level of cortisol in human mourning (Section 11.8). This pattern of release is also difficult to accomodate in our conventional view of emotions as relatively brief changes in state (but see Chapter 12). The pituitary–adrenal system, however, can produce hormonal release which is fairly brief and which occurs in the context of what we would normally wish to term emotional reactions.

Under these circumstances the release of adrenaline, noradrenaline and corticosterone is fairly specific. For example, Brady (1975*a*) has shown that a stimulus which elicits conditioned fear produces a release of both noradrenaline and corticosterone (but not adrenaline). Shock by itself does not cause release of either noradrenaline (Brady, 1975*a*) or corticosterone (Brady, 1975*b*) and hence the changes can be related specifically to the presence of conditioned as opposed to unconditioned fear (see Chapter 9 for discussion of this distinction).

Such studies also suggest that the relationship between the release of hormones and the extent to which the control of behaviour can be termed emotional is close. For example, Brady (1975*b*) reports increases in the release of corticosterone which parallel to a large extent the development of conditioned suppression in the same animals. In conditioned suppression, the animal is faced with a stimulus which predicts the delivery of an inescapable shock. After a number of pairings of stimulus and shock, presentation of the stimulus will suppress ongoing responding such as pressing a lever in order to obtain food. This suppression occurs despite the fact that the animal loses food by not responding and despite the fact that the change in responding does not affect the delivery of shock. This conditioned suppression is usually taken as an indication of fear in the animal (see Chapter 9). Since the shock is inescapable we might expect, intuitively, that the animal would remain 'afraid' throughout training, and corticosterone levels certainly remain high. Similarly, Coover, Ursin & Levine (1973) showed that plasma corticosterone levels were markedly above baseline during the initial acquisition of an avoidance response, i.e. in a task where the animal initially receives shocks but can avoid them if it makes the appropriate response. They also found that corticosterone levels decreased back towards baseline as avoidance learning approached and reached asymptote, i.e. as successful responding prevented the occurrence of any shock, when, intuitively we might expect the animal to have no further reason to be 'afraid'. These different patterns of results in conditioned suppression and avoidance tasks suggest that corticosterone release was the result of emotion since *all* the observed changes in level of corticosterone were paralleled by similar changes in the amount of defecation (see Gray, 1987, for the justification of defecation as a measure of fear). The pattern of release of corticosterone is also essentially the same as that shown when conditioned suppression is used to assess the level of fear produced by the discriminative stimulus in an avoidance experiment (Kamin, Brimer & Black, 1963). In the experiment of Coover *et al.* (1973), the release of corticosterone was shown not to result simply from the delivery of shock because it increased again when the animals were faced with forced extinction, i.e. when they were prevented from making the avoidance response, but did not receive shock. Likewise, the release of corticosterone could not be attributed simply to the fact that learning was taking place since there was no equivalent increase in corticosterone during the acquisition of an appetitive response, when a similar response was being learned but when food rather than shock was being used as the reinforcer (Coover, Goldman & Levine, 1971).

However, the corticosterone response is not specific to fear since it also occurs, for example, during the extinction of appetitive responding when frustration (see Chapter 7) rather than fear would be operative (Coover, Goldman & Levine, 1971). This result is particularly important since corticosterone is released in response to a wide variety of stressors as part of the General Adaptation Syndrome proposed by Selye (see Gray, 1987; Hoyenga & Hoyenga, 1984; for reviews). Many of the manipulations which are used to generate stress are also likely to induce fear, but it may be that some do not. The results with frustration show that fear is not a necessary condition for the release of corticosterone (Note 5.1).

We may, therefore, draw two conclusions about the release of hormones during emotion. First, hormonal release is not a nonspecific general concomitant of activation of the animal or of learning. Secondly, despite this, the release of a hormone need not be specific to one single emotion (fear versus frustration in the above examples). Both of these conclusions are consistent with the supposed teleonomy of such hormonal release in terms of making the animal ready for certain types of action. Specific emotions may share requirements for action with some emotions but not others.

5.7.   Emotion-specific changes in autonomic response

The autonomic nervous system has often been seen as providing a diffuse control of sympathetic tone. However, the varied innervation provided by the autonomic nervous system suggests that internal physiological response is unlikely to be a unitary reaction which is simply greater or lesser in magnitude on different occasions. Recently it has become clear that 'the sympathetic nervous system can be seen to be a highly differentiated, rapidly activated system, with subdivisions specialized to regulate different organ functions in response to the changing demands of the external and internal milieu' (Wallin & Fagius, 1986, p.63).

There is considerable evidence that different emotional states can be accompanied by different patterns of peripheral changes. The earliest and most cited study of this sort is that of Ax (1953). He elicited fear in subjects by implying that there was a potentially lethal short circuit in his recording apparatus and he elicited anger by the use of insult by the experimenter. (His methods were highly effective, but would not be considered ethical nowadays!) He found that there were changes in a wide variety of variables. Fear and anger produced equivalent changes in face temperature, heart output volume and systolic blood pressure. Anger produced greater changes than fear in galvanic skin response, heart rate, general muscle tension and diastolic blood pressure; while fear produced greater changes than anger in *peaks* of muscle tension and respiration rate. Schachter (1957) used virtually identical methods and indeed some of the same subjects as Ax. He also added a condition in which pain was induced by having the subjects place their hands into an ice bucket. He obtained similar results to Ax and in addition found that he could differentiate pain from either fear or anger on the basis of peripheral resistance to blood flow, which was increased in pain, decreased by fear and unaffected by anger, while a variety of other measures, affected by both fear and anger were not affected by pain.

Ax suggested that the changes in response to fear were due to adrenaline release, while the changes in response to anger were due to noradrenaline release. Funkenstein (1955) has extended this general idea to a differentiation of clinical patients on the basis of whether heart rate changes are dependent on adrenaline or noradrenaline and has suggested that the different species-specific tendencies of lions and rabbits are related to the high levels of adrenaline in the former and of noradrenaline in the latter!

Further studies have investigated similar variables to those measured by Ax finding reasonably distinctive changes in sadness and mirth (Averill, 1969), in sexual arousal resulting from reading sexually stimulating material (Wenger, Averill & Smith, 1968) and during the solution of intellectual problems (Stanners, Coulter, Sweet & Murphy, 1979). Differing patterns of autonomic change have also been reported with simple posing of different emotional facial expressions (Ekman, Levenson & Friesen, 1983; see also Chapter 10). The possi-

Table 5.1. *Relative variations in different aspects of cardiovascular change accompanying different emotions (Ax, 1953; Averill, 1969; Wenger, Averill & Smith, 1968; Roberts & Weerts, 1982).*

Note that, while no particular measure in itself distinguishes one emotion from another, the pattern across the 3 measures is distinctive. Symbols in the table are: + increase; ++ large increase; 0 no effect; – decrease.

	Heart rate	Systolic blood pressure	Diastolic blood pressure
fear	+	+	+
anger	++	+	++
sadness	–	+	+
mirth	+	0	0
sex	0	+	+

bility of differentiating the emotions is shown, using only cardiovascular measures, in Table 5.1.

Many other measures besides cardiovascular ones are routinely collected in such experiments; and very many more remain to be measured (especially in relation to the effects of hormonal release). It seems likely, therefore, that a high degree of differentiation between many emotions will be possible. However, some care needs to be taken in making comparisons. It is possible, for example, that at least some of the differences in pattern seen in Table 5.1 are simply the result of failure to equate the intensities of the different emotions felt. Thus, fear might be easier to obtain at high intensity in an experimental situation than anger – and noradrenaline might only be released with high intensities of emotion. For example, Levi (1965) investigated peripheral responses to humour and to tragedy and found similar patterns of response, except with large anxious reactions. Kety has suggested an alternative possibility: that adrenaline is secreted in situations of uncertainty while noradrenaline is secreted in situations where the outcome is certain. In my opinion the nature of the variations within Table 5.1, and more especially in the other items measured in the various studies, are difficult to account for in this way. However, it is clear that more careful 'dose–response' curves need to be obtained to be conclusive. For example, Roberts and Weerts (1982) used imagery techniques to produce individually tailored scenes designed for each subject to be neutral or to provoke low or high levels of anger or fear. Neutral scenes produced negligible cardiovascular responses. At low intensity, fear and anger produced similar increases in diastolic pressure, systolic pressure and heart rate. However, at high intensity, fear produced less of an increase in diastolic pressure than it had at low intensity whereas all other measures for fear and all measures for anger showed larger increases than at low intensity.

Another factor which is important when comparing results from one experiment to another is that the basic pattern of changes seen, particularly in the cardiovascular system, may change with apparently extraneous features of the testing situation – as, for example, whether the subjects are encouraged to move or not when expressing the emotion (Schwarz, Weinberger & Singer, 1981). Likewise, although pupillary changes often accompany cardiovascular changes, the former are controlled more by the cognitive demands of a task and the latter by non-cognitive factors (Stanners, Coulter, Sweet & Murphy, 1979). Finally, a point which is as important with animal experiments as human, we need to be sure that the imposed stimulus manipulation is in fact generating the intended emotion, and is producing essentially the same state in all subjects (e.g. Funkenstein, King & Drolette, 1954). Equally, our view of the likely teleonomy of autonomic changes is unlike James's original hypothesis in that we need not presume that feelings are the only things differentiating emotions. It is, therefore, relatively unimportant if some emotions are accompanied by similar peripheral patterns, provided that the feelings associated with those patterns are also similar (Note 5.2).

5.8.   Do visceral reactions determine what emotion is reported?

I have argued that peripheral feedback is necessary for the feeling component of emotion. Data discussed in the next chapter suggest that it is also important for the normal course of learning, at least of avoidance responses. In the previous section I have argued that there are differences in peripheral response between some emotions, but it is clear that, especially if intensity of emotion is controlled, there may also be strong similarities (Levi, 1965). Even if there are differences that the scientist can detect in such patterns, they need not be differences which are critical determinants of the specific emotion perceived by the subject. It is entirely possible, on the data reviewed so far, that peripheral feedback determines whether an emotion is accompanied by feelings but does not of itself determine *which* emotion is felt.

One of Cannon's criticisms of James was that artificial induction of visceral changes did not produce emotion. It is certainly true that such changes do not do so when induced by simple injections of, say, adrenaline. However, one reason for this finding could well be the simplicity of the technique used. If there are variations in peripheral change due to differential release by different emotions of a variety of humoural agents then injection of a single compound will not duplicate the peripheral changes associated with any emotion. Our discussion of the adrenal hormones shows this and it is likely to be true of other systems as well. A second reason for negative findings is that the temporal pattern of release of a compound into the blood stream in response to a stimulus could well differ from the pattern produced by an injection, and this pattern could then relate to specific effects on interacting target organs. More importantly, even if we restrict ourselves to autonomic reactions it is worth noting that injections of adrenaline can at best mimic changes produced by autonomic innervation of the adrenals and completely bypass the effects which can be presumed to occur in other autonomic target organs. Given these points it is hardly surprising that simple injections of adrenaline are not usually reported to induce identifiable emotions. In fact, it seems surprising to me that anyone should have expected that they would. However, even in the main study quoted by Cannon as negative evidence, some subjects did report normal emotions in response to injections of adrenaline.

A lack of reports of emotional changes could also relate to the method of questioning. Thus, Cantrill & Hunt (1932) found that injections of adrenaline caused subjects to say that they felt *as if* they were afraid or angry, or to say that they thought they would be susceptible to emotional suggestions. So, it is entirely possible that, even in subjects who did not report emotion proper, the drugs were producing feelings identical or very similar to those which would have accompanied an emotion. So, while it is clear that manipulation of peripheral physiological state is not sufficient to generate emotion, it could generate isolated feelings which could become integrated with other emotional influences.

How could such integration occur? Schachter & Singer (1962) provide an answer to this in a paper which has been extensively quoted, although not always in a complimentary manner (e.g. Plutchik & Ax, 1967; Zimbardo, Ebbesen & Maslach, 1977). Schachter & Singer gave injections of adrenaline to subjects who were either informed about the effects of the drug or kept in ignorance of its effects. The subjects were then exposed to stooges purporting to be other subjects in the experiment who acted in ways intended to produce either euphoria or anger. The result reported was that the injections produced the appropriate emotion provided that the subjects did not know the expected effects of the drug.

This result has been rather difficult to replicate, particularly with respect to the bidirectional nature of the emotions induced. Even when bidirectionality has been obtained, the results have not always conformed to theory. For example, Erdman & Janke (1978), who report one of the successful replications with manipulations of 'anger' and 'happiness', nonetheless found that changes in an additional 'anxiety' condition were not as expected. As far as generation of aversive emotion is concerned, the results are more promising. Lader & Tyrer (1975) conclude that for a number of studies

the differences in the results of later workers are explicable in retrospect by the presence or absence of anxiety-provoking environmental cues. In a neutral setting the injection of epinephrine (adrenaline) produced no emotional changes, 'cold emotion', or 'as if' emotion .... In an anxiety-provoking setting, intentionally or accidentally created by the experimenters, subjects showed more evidence of anxiety and in a minority of cases panic attacks were elicited.

(op. cit.)

The effects of injections of adrenaline on avoidance behaviour in rats seem to be consistent with this (e.g. Latane & Schachter, 1962; see also Pare, 1969, for a discussion of dose levels). Similarly, Maslach (1979) reports that in an exact replication of the Schachter & Singer experiment, Marshall found that intense peripheral changes produced a unpleasant emotional state independent of the stooge condition. She also carried out a variant of the basic experiment in which hypnosis rather than injection was used to change the subject's state of arousal; again unexplained arousal resulted in reports of unpleasant emotions independent of whether the stooge was happy or not (although their behaviour towards the 'happy' stooge was sociable).

Schachter & Wheeler (1962) provide one of the few reports of successful manipulation of pleasant emotions. They used a comic film rather than a stooge to manipulate their subjects and found that injections of adrenaline, which would have been expected to produce 'unexplained arousal', increased overt amusement, e.g. laughing. By contrast, chlorpromazine, a major tranquilliser which Schachter & Wheeler argued would decrease arousal decreased amusement. However, their positive results were obtained only on scores of overt amusement during the film as assessed by external observers. The subjects' self reports after the film were not affected in the same way. They obtained comments such as 'I couldn't understand why I was laughing during the movie'. A case of an 'as if' skeletal response, perhaps?

At this stage of the evidence, it seems we can accept the idea that peripheral changes can result in reports of emotions which would not have occurred, or which would not have been so intense, in the absence of such changes. Given the studies which have shown distinct patterns of peripheral responses in different emotions we might also expect that specific peripheral changes would result in specific emotions. However, failures to replicate Schachter & Singer's experiment could be due to the fact that a laboratory experiment is likely to involve aversive stimuli. Instruction to a stooge to 'act happy' may or may not, therefore, result in a pleasant effect. More importantly, injection of a single compound could well produce peripheral changes which are a common subset of the changes normally found in a variety of emotions. The exact relationship between the pattern of peripheral change, cognitive state and emotion must be viewed as unresolved, especially when there may be a distinction between the presence of emotion and verbal reports of emotion.

If more experiments such as these are to be performed it seems to me important that they should be undertaken with great care to maintain a natural context, both psychological and physiological. If the various hypotheses are to be properly tested then injections should consist of the correct mixture of as many as possible of the compounds which are normally released by *that particular subject* in different emotions (at the least noradrenaline should be compared to or mixed with adrenaline). Also, injection should be arranged in such a way (e.g. via an indwelling catheter) that the subject is unaware that it is taking place and in such a way that the amounts of the compounds released into the bloodstream have a time course in relation to any stimuli used which matches the time course of their release in response to natural emotion-releasing stimuli. Finally, great care is required in choice of stimuli and the situation in which they are presented. Stooges may or may not be able to generate the desired emotion in a subject depending both on their acting ability and on the extent to which the laboratory situation biases interpretation of the stooge's behaviour. Likewise, a photograph of Ronald Reagan may incline some to laugh but others to cry. In some respects commercial horror and comedy films might be a good choice, aimed as they are at a mass audience, especially since the testing situation could be under good control without being a laboratory. Even here, however, one is likely to obtain idiosyncratic responses to the material (see interview data in Schachter & Wheeler, 1962).

5.9.   Conclusion

We have, therefore, evidence that physiological changes can contribute to the feeling component of emotion – and may in fact represent a major part of emotional feelings. It is also clear that different patterns of autonomic and hormonal response occur in different emotions. It is not yet clear how far specific patterns of somatic response determine the specific feelings which accompany an emotion. Schachter's experiments, described in the present chapter also suggest that somatic changes can result in changes in cognitive and other aspects of emotion. This is a more contentious issue, with which we will deal in the next chapter.

6: Somatic influences on the emotions

The restless violence of the senses impetuously carries away the mind of even a wise man striving towards perfection

Bhagavad Gita: 2-60

6.1. Do physiological changes determine emotion?

Introspection suggests that we perceive some fact and evaluate it; that this evaluation results in an emotional state which causes us to act; and that this emotional state is then accompanied or followed by specific feelings. As was discussed in Chapter 1, James (1884) suggested 'on the contrary ... that the bodily changes follow directly the perception of the exciting fact, and that our feelings of the same changes as they occur *is* the emotion' and this has been taken to imply that emotional behaviour would not occur in the absence of feeling.

Cannon (1927) proposed a number of objections to James's position which are at the heart of much of the research we will discuss:

1. Total separation of the viscera from the CNS does not alter emotional behaviour.
2. The same visceral changes occur in very different emotional states and in non-emotional states.
3. The viscera are relatively insensitive structures.
4. Visceral changes are too slow to be the source of emotional feeling.
5. Artificial induction of the visceral changes typical of strong emotions does not produce them.

As we will see, there appears to be some truth in each of these suggestions, but in each case they do not represent the entire truth. In effect, despite the fact that their views are often represented as being opposed to each other, we will find that James and Cannon each appear to be equally right (or wrong).

6.2. Effects of peripheral sympathectomy

While not as conclusive a test of the role of peripheral feedback as the total sensory denervation of paraplegics discussed in the previous chapter, peripheral sympathectomy, the surgical destruction of peripheral sympathetic nerves, provides a test which can be used in behaving animals. Peripheral sympathectomy prevents the normal occurrence of a variety of bodily changes and hence, *a fortiori*, prevents sensory feedback of those changes. It would also remove specifically visceral feedback of bodily sensations (see Cervero & Sharkey, 1985) – it would not, however, remove proprioceptive feedback of muscular and other changes produced by hormonal release (Figure 5.1). As Cannon suggests, a variety of authors have reported that emotional behaviour does not seem to change in animals which have been subjected to peripheral sympathectomy. So not all aspects of emotion depend on peripheral autonomic feedback. However, the discussions of teleonomy in Chapters 2 and 3 suggest that in considering the releasing properties of emotion we may have to deal independently with the release of simple skeletal responses and the release of feelings. Even if the latter are not, as is shown by the data, causally antecedent to skeletal responses, they may none the less affect them.

Wynne & Solomon (1955) performed an experiment which bears on this and has often been cited in support of Cannon's position. However, in the context of our present question a closer look at their data is warranted. They tested dogs which had received surgical peripheral sympathectomies (Figure 5.1). The dogs were tested for acquisition and performance of an avoidance response – pressing a panel in order to avoid a shock. Both groups of animals came to perform the avoidance response with equal efficiency, and animals lesioned after learning the response retained it perfectly even when tested 5 months later. An important finding was that the groups did in fact differ in their rate of *acquisition* of avoidance. In Chapter 9 we discuss data which show that fear, as indexed by conditioned suppression or by defecation, occurs only during the initial acquisition of the avoidance response, as indeed does release of corticosterone (see Chapter 5). In fact Wynne and Solomon themselves conclude that painful or fear provoking stimuli result in autonomic nervous system discharge, skeletal responses, and hormonal responses and that all three of these can result in feedback stimuli to the animal. Thus, the data from Wynne & Solomon's experiment provide some support for Cannon's position in that learning of an avoidance response can occur, albeit slowly, in the absence of peripheral feedback (i.e. motivation *per se* does not depend on feeling). The data also suggest, however, that James may be partially right in that peripheral feedback does contribute to emotion as measured by the *acquisition* of avoidance (see Chapter 9 for a discussion of whether emotion is involved in the performance of positively and negatively reinforced responses).

This is, of course, essentially the same conclusion as was drawn from the observations of humans with various levels of spinal lesion (Section 5.4).

6.3.   Non-surgical manipulation of the sympathetic system

All of the above data were based on human or infrahuman subjects with transected neural pathways. More recently the technique of immunosympathectomy has been employed to reduce peripheral feedback. In this procedure the experimenter injects an agent which causes the selective loss of sympathetic nerves through immune reactions. Occasionally such studies appear to show impaired acquisition of avoidance (Wenzel & Jeffrey, 1967) but more generally they find no changes in avoidance, or defecation or other measures such as food reinforced lever pressing (Wenzel & Nagle, 1965; see Van Toller & Tarpy, 1974 for review). Unfortunately, these studies suffer from a number of flaws. While the immunosympathectomy technique is highly sophisticated, the behavioural data presented tend to be unclear. The performance of the avoidance response is reported with little care in the following of acquisition. In one case, for example, the acquisition data presented show no evidence of improved responding in control animals with trials (Van Toller & Tarpy, 1972), which makes it difficult to conclude that any learning was involved at all. Finally, and most seriously there are problems with the immunosympathectomy technique itself: the lesion often leaves as much as 30% of the sympathetic system intact (e.g. Wenzel & Nagle, 1965) and although it can get as low as 10% (Wenzel, 1968) its effects are never total. Thus neither the positive, nor the negative, results reported appear conclusive. A further consideration is that the manipulation is carried out while the animals are very young and that negative results, even with improved technique, might not be particularly meaningful in relation to the behaviour of the normal adult animal.

By contrast, drugs which act to reduce sympathetic nervous activity have clear effects on behaviour. Some of the drugs have effects on both central and peripheral nervous activity but it is their peripheral effects that seems most important. These drugs have been investigated for specifically anxiolytic activity. As we would expect from our discussion of the role of peripheral systems the drugs are not anxiolytic in the most general sense (see introduction to Salmon & Gray, 1986). Rather, they appear to be most effective in anxiety states which have a strong peripheral component. This conclusion is exemplified in a study by Neftel & coworkers (1982) employing a natural source of anxiety.

Some musicians suffer from stage fright to an extent which can impair their performance. Neftel *et al.* studied a group of musicians who received either a peripheral autonomic blocking agent or placebo before performing either in the presence or in the absence of an audience. The placebo group showed a significant impairment of technical performance when playing in front of an audience. The drug group showed a slight, non-significant, improvement. The drug also produced a significant reduction in ratings of stage fright as assessed by a specially devised questionnaire. Animal studies have also shown that, while such blocking agents can affect behaviour in a manner similar to that of conventional anxiolytic drugs, especially when they are administered acutely, they only do so in a limited range of circumstances (Salmon & Gray, 1985*a,b*, 1986).

The conclusion from human paraplegic studies (Section 5.4) was that peripheral feedback appears to be necessary for at least some aspects of reported feelings – and hence may be an important generator of feelings. The conclusion from animal experiments is that such feedback is important at least for the acquisition of avoidance behaviour. Both human and animal data show that peripheral feedback is not necessary for the demonstration of emotional behaviour. Both human and animal data also show that peripheral reactions can influence emotional behaviour. These data are consistent with a weak form of James's position: that feelings play an active role in emotion rather than merely being a passive consequence of it. Equally, as suggested by Cannon, peripheral feedback does not seem to be essential for the eventual acquisition of avoidance behaviour in animals nor for the skeletal components of expression of a variety of emotions in humans.

6.4.   Emotion after the removal of hormonal influences

As was mentioned in Section 5.3, the release of corticosterone (or cortisol in humans) from the adrenal cortex is produced by the release of ACTH from the pituitary. Thus, in most situations ACTH and corticosterone will both be present, in varying amounts and with differing time courses. If we remove the adrenals, we will prevent the release of corticosterone without preventing the release of ACTH – in fact, levels of ACTH will increase as corticosterone normally inhibits its release through negative feedback. If we remove the pituitary, we will, essentially, prevent release of both hormones. Both glands release a variety of other substances and so, if we wish to show that the effects of removal of the gland are due to loss of one specific compound, it is necessary to reinstate that compound by exogenous administration. Experiments with hormones have, therefore, been more complicated than those with sympathectomy described in the previous sections. A final problem is that adrenalectomy removes not only the adrenal cortex but also the adrenal medulla and few experimenters have looked at the effects of medullectomy in its own right.

Manipulation of the pituitary–adrenal system has a variety of effects on behaviour, particularly avoidance behaviour (Note 6.1). Injection of corticosterone, where it has been tested, reverses the effects of adrenalectomy. It should not be assumed, however, that the results of adrenalectomy are therefore due to loss of corticosterone in the first place since there is a negative feedback relationship between corticosterone and ACTH. Thus changes in extinction of avoidance, for example, observed with adrenalectomy could be due to either low levels of corticosterone or high levels of ACTH. Additional removal of the pituitary in adrenalectomised animals produces extinction comparable to that of intact control animals; suggesting that in this case a high level of ACTH is the critical factor. The data are complex, but a number of simple suggestions can be derived from them. First, it appears that the pituitary–adrenal system is involved in at least some aspects of avoidance learning. This does not appear to be due to involvement of the adrenal medulla, and the results of Moyer & Bunnell (1959) suggest that the effects of peripheral sympathectomy on the acquisition of avoidance learning (Wynne & Solomon, 1955) are independent of the adrenals. Autonomic and hormonal influences may well play separate, complementary roles in relation to avoidance. One might expect that loss of *both* autonomic and hormonal influences would have much more extensive effects than the sum of their individual effects (Note 6.2).

Secondly, it is clear that the release of ACTH is important in affecting avoidance behaviour independently of its effects in releasing corticosterone. Given the fact that ACTH is released as an initial response to many situations and that corticosterone may only reach high levels some time later, we could expect somewhat different roles for the two hormones. It may well be that many of the correlations of corticosterone level with behavioural condition reflect a role not of corticosterone itself but of ACTH, with corticosterone merely acting as a marker for ACTH. However, it seems likely that corticosterone, while having both a feedback function on ACTH release and having peripheral metabolic functions, also has a direct influence on behaviour.

Thirdly, the actions of the adrenal medulla, the adrenal cortex and the autonomic nervous system are likely to be coordinated. Moyer

(1958*b*) points out that 'the secretions of the (adrenal) cortex tend to have a facilitative effect on the autonomic nervous system ... . At the same time the medullary secretion has a depressing effect'. Thus secretions of both the adrenal cortex and the adrenal medulla feedback in a negative fashion on their own release and may well interact with each other in a positive fashion. Such organisation would produce a well regulated activity in both systems which would be synchronised to some extent.

6.5.   Secretions of the pituitary–adrenal cortex as controllers of emotion

Experiments with exogenous administration of hormones other than adrenaline have usually been carried out in the context of animal learning experiments rather than human report or behaviour. As before, we will restrict consideration of the effects of exogenous administration of hormones to the actions of ACTH and corticosterone.

As noted above, there is a positive relationship between the release of ACTH and the release of corticosterone and a negative feedback relationship between the release of corticosterone and the release of ACTH. Exogenous administration of ACTH is therefore accompanied by an increase in corticosterone, while exogenous administration of corticosterone is accompanied by a reduction in circulating ACTH.

Consideration of experiments which separate these interacting effects (Note 6.3) leads to a similar conclusion from the effects of exogenous administration of pituitary adrenal hormones as our conclusions from the effects of adrenalectomy: that we must be prepared for a role of both ACTH and corticosterone in behaviour related to both fear and frustration. The extent to which these compounds induce as opposed to modulate emotion is unclear. It does appear to be the case, however, that they are not involved in appetitive behaviour. This would tend to argue against Schachter & Singer's (1962) position, since differences in the patterns of substances released in any particular emotion increase the chance that it is a particular pattern which results in the report by the subject of a particular emotion or emotional feeling.

6.6.   False feedback experiments

The previous sections discussed experiments which attempted to change emotions by manipulating peripheral physiological state. In discussing their original results, Schachter & Singer (1962) proposed that the perception of such changes produces a need to evaluate the situation in an emotional way. This raises the question of whether it is the perception of such changes or merely their presence which could be affecting emotional judgements.

An attempt to answer this is provided by 'false feedback' experiments in which subjects are provided with feedback of what is, for example, supposed to be their own heart rate. They then perform a task and the effect of false, experimenter controlled, changes in the feedback are observed. Valins (1967) found that such false feedback of heart rate could affect judgement of the erotic quality of photographs, and Valins & Ray (1967) found equivalent changes in the observed fear reactions to snakes.

Although the results of these experiments are both interesting and replicable, there are problems with taking them at face value in relation to the normal control of emotion. For example, Truax (1983 – see this paper also for a brief review of false feedback studies) provided subjects with beeps which they were either told was feedback of heart rate or were told was feedback of galvanic skin response. The latter form of false feedback was just as effective as the former in modifying the subjects' perceptions, but *only if* the subject had previously been informed as to the functional nature of galvanic skin response. This result shows that the effects of false feedback are not dependent on any similarity between the nature of the false feedback and the nature of the changes which supposedly supply normal feedback; nor are the effects dependent on stimulus change; rather the effects appear to be occurring at a purely cognitive level.

There are other methodological problems. Goldstein, Fink & Mettee (1972) found that the delivery of false heart rate feedback changes the actual heart rate. Valins's results might be due, then, not to perception of false changes but to an effect, perceived or otherwise, of actual changes. Worse is to come. Mandler & Kahn (1960) found that subjects could not in general perceive their own heart rate. They performed two experiments in which subjects had to indicate changes in their own heart rate by responding either verbally or by moving a lever. Subjects could not perform the task when they were given feedback as to whether responses were correct or incorrect, but were not told that it was based on heart rate changes. They could perform the task when they were told that it was based on heart rate but, even then, their success depended on adjusting their breathing patterns so as to control their heart rate, rather than on detection of the heart rate itself.

6.7.   A role for heart rate changes

Although not strictly relevant to the question of the role of the perception of heart rate or other physiological changes in themselves, the
false-feedback data imply that *if* a subject could perceive changes in
their heart rate this could well affect their emotional state, or at least
their judgement of it. Schandry (1981) investigated the accuracy of
perception of cardiac response in a number of subjects. Thus, he
required subjects to estimate their heart rates (without being allowed
to take their own pulse). He then divided his subjects into a group of
'good perceivers' and a group of 'poor perceivers'. The former had
higher scores on scales of state anxiety (i.e. current anxiety as opposed
to trait anxiety which would reflect a long term personality characteristic) and emotional lability but did not differ significantly on actual
heart rate. (Scores on the so called Autonomic Perception Questionnaire did not appear to be related to actual cardiac perception.)

Sirota, Schwartz & Shapiro (1974, 1976) obtained comparable results in a different way. They administered a questionnaire (rather
than a direct test) on the basis of which they divided subjects into
'cardiac aware' and 'cardiac nonaware' groups. They then took subgroups of each of these groups and trained one subgroup to produce
voluntary increases in their heart rate and the other to produce voluntary decreases. Following training, the subjects were asked to assess
the painfulness of an electric shock. Cardiac aware subjects reported
the most extreme reponses – those trained to increase heart rate
reported high levels of pain, those trained to decrease it reported low
levels. Cardiac unaware subjects were intermediate in their reports of
pain and showed little effect of the training on their assessment of pain.

These data suggest that in the general population emotional judgements are not necessarily affected by changes in, for example, heart
rate. However, such changes may be influential in those persons who
are particularly aware of them. It is worth noting a problem with a
large amount of the research in this area – excessive reliance on
questionnaires. To my mind a questionnaire intended to assess perception of peripheral changes is superfluous when the exact accuracy of
such perception can be tested directly. Similarly, the effects of manipulations are frequently judged solely on the basis of answers to
questionnaires. This is fine if all we wish to assess is any change in
self-report. But changes in self-report need not be accompanied,
necessarily, by any change in behaviour and, equally, changes in
emotional behaviour need not be accompanied by changes in self-
report (Riskind & Gotay, 1982). In the context of the present book the

questionnaire has another major failing – you cannot administer it to an animal other than human.

6.8. Conclusion

It appears that emotions can result in both autonomic and hormonal responses each of which could well supply the basis for feelings. The release of hormones (including adrenaline) has the capacity to modify emotional behaviour and reports of emotional feelings. However, it is clear that the mere presence of any particular somatic change does not by itself result in emotion whatever its contribution to feelings. We can agree with Mandler (1984) that 'James's contribution is still important in that he led us to understand the relevance of autonomic arousal in the production of emotion, and Cannon's criticism is equally important in pointing out that emotions are *not* "nothing but" the perception of visceral arousal.' We may add that the same is likely to be true for the release of those hormones whose control owes nothing to the autonomic nervous system.

In one sense some of the data we have considered argue more strongly for a controlling role of feelings in emotion than appears at first sight. One of the main manipulations which has been used (injection of adrenaline) mimics neither the normal production of that compound, nor the normal pattern of other hormones which would accompany it, nor the outflow from the autonomic nervous system to target organs other than the adrenals. To have obtained any positive results at all is surprising. Likewise, given the data of Table 5.1, it seems entirely possible that the bidirectional effects suggested by Schachter & Singer could result from adrenaline producing a reaction which represents a common subset of the feelings which normally accompany a variety of emotions but which only weakly resembles the feelings of any one of them. A failure to duplicate this ambiguity sufficiently could, then, account for the reported failures to replicate the original result.

Not only do we need to keep in mind the complexity of autonomic and hormonal reactions which could contribute to feeling, but also we should be wary of concluding that peripheral physiological changes are the sole source of feelings. The stimuli resulting from a central emotional state could well depend purely on activity in the central nervous system via a form of reafference. More importantly, there is evidence that the peripheral feedback from, or possibly central reafference associated with, skeletal responses can also influence emotion. This is particularly true of facial expression which, in addition to direct proprioceptive effects, is capable of modifying autonomic activity (Chapter 10). Proprioception from facial and postural changes could also, of course, supply a component of emotional feeling (e.g. 'feeling tense'). It should be remembered also that many somatic changes in emotion (e.g. changes in red blood cells) need have no relation to feelings at all.

Given such a view of feelings we have one remaining problem. It is easy enough to see that the physiological changes which accompany emotion could have arisen through the type of selection pressure discussed by Cannon. It is also not unreasonable to suppose that sensory nerves, present to signal the state of a specific organ for some specific reason (e.g. signals of distension of the stomach to avoid dangerous overeating), would also signal changes in the equivalent organs produced by autonomic or hormonal action. Where such proprioception is distinctive it could obviously result in specific emotional feelings. However, it is by no means obvious why, teleonomically, such sensory information should have come to exert feedback control over an emotional state. This problem is addressed in the next chapter.

7: Optimal foraging and the partial reinforcement effect: a model for the teleonomy of feelings?

'Is there any other point to which you would wish to draw my attention?'
'To the curious incident of the dog in the night-time.'
'The dog did nothing in the night-time.'
'That was the curious incident,' remarked Sherlock Holmes
Arthur Conan-Doyle: Silver Blaze

7.1. Teleonomy, physiological change and feelings

Chapter 5 discussed a variety of physiological changes which can accompany emotions and which, we argued, adjust the organism's bodily systems in preparation for classes of action frequently required when that emotion is present. Chapter 6 concluded that such changes are not merely of physiological utility but can also play a controlling role in the psychology of emotion. As was noted, the presence of some compound such as adrenaline, or the changes in particular organ systems induced by such compounds, could come, through further evolution, to act as controllers of psychological states. *Why*, teleonomically speaking, they should do so is, however, not at all clear – and is quite likely to involve rather different reasons for different internal changes and different emotions.

In the present chapter I will discuss a particular behavioural phenomenon, the partial reinforcement extinction effect, and its underlying control. I will present a provisional account of the teleonomy of this phenomenon which will, I hope, show that reasonable teleonomic accounts of the psychological role of physiological changes can be constructed. There is, of course, no guarantee that any particular physiological change can be perceived, proprioceptively, by the organism concerned and so there need be no relation between such changes and feelings. However, in this case, the teleonomic argument hinges on the idea that the animal's emotional state can act as part of the normal stimulus complex controlling its behaviour – and so I have taken the liberty of using the word feeling in the title of the chapter. Likewise, there is no absolute guarantee that the stimuli referred to in the argument below necessarily result from the physiological changes which are known to occur – however, for the present it is parsimonious

77

to equate feelings with the perception of such changes. Thus, the argument presented here is intended as a *model* for equivalent arguments in relation to other phenomena and emotions rather than being conclusive in all respects. It is intended to show that the role of feelings *can* have a fairly straightforward teleonomy once basic control mechanisms have been delineated.

While straightforward the steps required in the argument are somewhat laborious. First, there is the assessment of the value of alternative strategies, theoretically available to the animal – and hence assessment of the functionality of the behaviour actually observed. Next, the mechanisms which generate the observed behaviour must be determined – and it turns out that there are several of these. Finally, the teleonomy of the individual mechanisms must be separately accounted for.

7.2.   How can you assess teleonomy of behaviour?

In addition to the reservations which I have just expressed about the status of the functional aspects of the arguments which follow, we must also be wary of the specifically teleonomic aspects. In previous chapters the adaptive value of, for example, reduced bleeding has been taken for granted. Even in these cases we have probably been somewhat cavalier in not considering possible costs to the animal of the physiological responses involved. (If there were no costs such as increased risk of thrombosis, it is difficult to see why a particular high level of clotting ability would not be maintained at all times.) In what follows, we must first consider the problem of defining what is appropriate, adaptive behaviour in particular circumstances.

In the case of working for food, which we will be considering below, the problem is to define what would be optimal feeding (or foraging) behaviour. Analysis of this type of problem has led to 'optimal foraging theory' which has been described as 'an attempt to understand the decision rules of foraging animals. The rationale of (optimal foraging theory) is that these decision rules have been shaped by natural selection to allow the animal to perform as efficiently as possible' (Krebs, Stephens & Sutherland, 1983, p.166). It should be noted, however, that the solution of a problem via optimality theory and the decision rules used by an animal solving the same problem are unlikely to bear any resemblance to each other. Equally, a variety of different 'optimal' solutions can be derived for any particular set of environmental conditions depending on the assumptions which are made at the outset. For

example, in considering rewards different authors have studied opti-
misation of:

1. The expected reward over some time interval of duration T ...
2. The average reward per unit time.
3. The expected discounted reward: where rewards incurred at time t in
   the future are discounted by a factor.

(McNamara & Houston, 1980)

Each of these optimality criteria will result in a different solution as
to what is optimal behaviour. It is also clear that different species faced
with the same nominal problem may be faced by differing physiological constraints which redefine what is optimal. As one particularly
obvious boundary condition, there is no point in making a choice
which will deliver the largest expected reward over some time interval
of duration T if you are going to starve to death while waiting for it to
arrive.

To emphasise the difference between the calculations of the theorist
and those of the animal in any particular situation it is useful to
distinguish between optimal foraging rules and 'rules of thumb'. For
example, the parasite *Nemeritis canescens* 'allocates its searching time
in relation to host density approximately as predicted by an optimal
foraging model (but) the decision rule used by *Nemeritis* ... is a simple
mechanism based on habituation to host scent – a far cry from the
Lagrange multipliers and Newton's iterative approximations used by
the theorist to solve the problem' (Krebs *et al.*, 1983, p.188).

One view of optimal foraging models of behaviour, then, is that they
provide an ideal limiting case to which the animal's inbuilt rules of
thumb can aspire – given that all of the relevant cost and benefit items
have been included in the theorist's calculations.

7.3. Optimality and the partial reinforcement extinction effect (PREE)

McNamara & Houston (1980) have addressed the 'general problem of
how long to persist when responses no longer yield rewards'. It can be
seen that this will be a common problem for animals. The bird collect-
ing worms from one 'patch' of the lawn will eventually deplete the
patch to the point where it would be wiser to move; the fisherman will
find that fish stop biting at certain times; and so on. The specific case
considered by McNamara & Houston is where, for a number of initial
responses, an animal receives a reward with some constant probability
p, and then, for subsequent responses, never receives a reward. It is

assumed that the making of a response incurs some cost to the animal. In one sense, optimal behaviour is easily defined: the animal should never make the response once reward is no longer available. In practice, the animal does not know when this has happened since chance runs of nonrewarded responding will occur during the rewarded period except when $p=1.0$. The optimality problem then becomes one of defining at what point one should be sufficiently certain that no further food is forthcoming to terminate responding, given the potential reward to be gained and the actual costs of continued responding.

Given known values of the gain from each reward, the cost of each response, the value of p, and the assumption of an optimality criterion of maximisation of the expected total reward minus costs McNamara & Houston calculated the number of nonrewarded responses an 'optimal' animal should make before ceasing to respond. They point out that their model is simplified in that, under realistic conditions, p will not be constant and will not be known by the animal – and one could add that, in some cases, the values of gain and cost will not be known exactly either. None the less, consideration of the effect that such changes would have shows that, 'regardless of the exact details, the optimal policy for this sort of problem involves persisting for more trials in the face of failure if p is low. This provides an explanation of the PREE in terms of optimality theory' (McNamara & Houston, 1980, p.687).

The PREE is relatively simple at the observational level. Two groups of animals are trained to make a response, such as running in an alley, for food. One group always receives reward (continuous reinforcement), the second group receives reward on only some trials (partial reinforcement). After the response is established both groups are put into extinction, that is to say they receive no further food. The continuously reinforced group will tend to stop responding during extinction before the partially reinforced group. This is the PREE.

The PREE is interesting in a number of ways. First, it is, as behavioural phenomena go, both very robust and very widespread phylogenetically (see Jenkins & Stanley, 1950; Lewis, 1960). Secondly, it shows that there is no simple relation between the strength of conditioned connections and the number of deliveries of the reward which is supposed to strengthen those connections. Suppose our two groups receive the same number of acquisition trials. If the partially reinforced group are on a 50% schedule, they will only receive half the number of rewards received by the continuously reinforced group. If response–reward pairings are all that is important they will have developed, therefore, only half the strength of the conditioned connections of the continuously rewarded group. The partial group might be expected, therefore, to show lesser resistance to extinction. What is 'predicted' by optimality theory and what is actually observed is the PREE: the partial group show greater resistance to extinction than the continuous group. The explanation of the PREE provided by McNamara & Houston (1980) is not the same general class of explanation, however, as would be provided by a reinforcement theorist. Optimality theory here does not provide a true prediction of what the animal will do but, instead, provides an estimate of adaptiveness of a particular kind of behaviour pattern which can be used in a teleonomic assessment of the behaviour. Indeed, they give in their paper a possible rule of thumb which would normally allow an animal to behave optimally. This involves a) remembering the number of non-rewarded trials which have occurred since the last rewarded response; b) remembering a weighting factor; and c) reducing the weighting factor whenever a run of non-rewarded trials is followed by reward. The decision rule is then to cease responding when the current number of non-rewarded trials multiplied by the current value of the weighting factor exceeds the amount of reward normally received. (This rule of thumb is in the same general 'nonemotional' class as the theory of Capaldi described below, but differs in that Capaldi assumes that the animal is sensitive to the pattern as well as the number of non-rewarded trials.) Mathematically this rule of thumb is simple to operate and in practice it will normally produce 'optimal' behaviour. Interestingly, there is one case where the rule departs from optimality: when a period of partial reinforcement is followed by a period of continuous reinforcement and this is in turn followed by extinction. The optimal behaviour, in terms of their model of optimality, would be speedy extinction but the rule of thumb they propose would lead to slow extinction – as it happens rats show slow extinction in this case!

We have, then, an optimality analysis which advocates persistence in the face of partial reinforcement; we have at least one possible simple rule of thumb which could generally generate such persistence; and we have the observation that animals do in general persist. The question arises: what rules do animals in fact use to generate their persistence? We will see that they use a variety of 'rules', some unrelated to emotion, some dependent on emotion and on the feelings which accompany emotion

7.4. Omission of reward and the generation of frustration

Before proceeding it will be necessary first to discuss the status of frustration in psychology in order to derive an objective basis for discussing it. It will also be necessary to distinguish between unconditioned and conditioned (i.e. anticipatory) frustration as these have rather different properties in terms of the control of behaviour. (It may be remembered that hormonal and autonomic reactions also vary depending on whether conditioned or unconditioned reactions are being considered.)

Mackintosh (1974, pp.305–6) remarks on the reluctance of learning theorists to attribute properties to events which do not occur. A non-event would certainly not be expected to have consequences. However, there is a world of difference between no occurrence at all of some event and the omission of an event which has previously occurred regularly. This point is brought out objectively by an experiment carried out by Amsel & Roussel (1952).

Amsel & Roussel trained hungry rats to run in a double runway which had two goal boxes, one in the middle of the runway and one at the end. The rats were always rewarded in the end goal box. In the middle box, the rats sometimes received food and sometimes did not. They found that the rats ran faster in the second runway after omission of reward in the middle goal box than after reward. This effect is not due simply to a higher level of hunger after non-reward than after reward. Control rats, who never receive reward in the middle goal box, run slower than do the experimental rats after reward and even run slower than rats who always receive reward in the middle goal box (Wagner, 1959). Thus omission of an expected reward has effects unlike those of total non-occurrence of reward.

The double runway demonstrates a changed state in the animal as a result of omission of an expected reward. What are the properties of this state?

In one sense, the increased speed in the second part of the double runway can be viewed as the result of a releasing property of reward omission (Note 7.1). A clearer example of this type of effect is seen in the release of aggression. When a rat has just experienced omission of reward then it will display considerable aggression towards any other rat unlucky enough to be in its vicinity (Gallup, 1965). Similarly, a stimulus that has been paired with the omission of reward can subsequently potentiate a startle response to a separate stimulus (Wagner, 1963); and such a stimulus produces nearly as great an increase in subsequent rearing and movement within an open field as does omission of reward itself (Gallup & Hare, 1969). Thus both unconditioned states resulting from reward omission, and conditioned states resulting from stimuli which have been paired with reward omission, can help release behaviour in an energising fashion (Hinde, 1966, pp.88–9) when appropriate releasing stimuli (see, e.g. Konishi, 1971) are present. I will refer to these states below as states of conditioned and unconditioned frustration (Note 7.2).

7.5.   Accounts of the PREE in terms of frustration

The notion of frustration as an aversive emotion (Note 7.1) can provide us with a simple explanation of the PREE. As discussed by Gray, Holt & McNaughton (1983), a PREE could theoretically result from a simple non-associative process – the development of a general tolerance to aversive events. They note that

a single session of inescapable shock impairs the rat's subsequent ability to learn escape or avoidance responses in a shuttle box; but the disruptive effect of inescapable shock disappeared if the rats were preexposed to 15 sessions rather than one such session. Thus repeated exposure to inescapable shock allows the rat to overcome the deleterious effects of a single session of inescapable shock. Miller (1976) has termed this effect toughening up. Toughening up has been shown by Chen & Amsel (1977) also to affect extinction of rewarded behaviour: inescapable shock prior to runway training (for food) increased subsequent resistance to extinction.

(Gray, Holt & McNaughton, 1983)

The shocks in Chen & Amsel's experiment were all delivered before any experience of reward and were delivered in a different apparatus from that used for runway training. The increased resistance to extinction observed must, therefore, have been the result of a non-associative process. We can account for the PREE in a similar manner. During acquisition the animal experiences frustration a number of times. This repeated aversive experience produces toughening up, which then, as in Chen & Amsel's experiment with shock, produces increased resistance to extinction.

Amsel (e.g.1967) provides a different account of the PREE in terms of frustration in which the critical assumption is that the state of conditioned frustration involves a detectable stimulus. During acquisition of running under partial reinforcement, unconditioned frustration (the immediate reaction to omission of an expected reward) follows the experience of apparatus cues and so conditioning can occur. On subsequent trials, these cues, as a result of the conditioning, can elicit a state of conditioned (anticipatory) frustration. On a 50% schedule of reinforcement this conditioned frustration will frequently be followed by reward. This pairing of the stimuli of conditioned frustration with reward will result in the conditioning of running to these stimuli.

Let us now see what transpires during extinction. Continuously reinforced animals, on receiving omission of reward, will experience unconditioned and after a few trials conditioned frustration. The aversive nature of conditioned frustration will reduce responding. This is an active reduction over and above a loss of responding through simple lack of reinforcement. By contrast, the partially reinforced animals are used to running in response to the stimuli of conditioned frustration and will continue, therefore, to run. Hence the PREE.

7.6.   Simple associative accounts of the PREE

Early accounts of the PREE did not postulate the involvement of emotions such as frustration, nor do some more recent theories.

Sutherland (1964) explains the PREE in terms of his theory of discrimination learning. This theory rests on the concept of an analyser. This is essentially equivalent to the type of feature extraction unit which neurophysiological and behavioural data suggest underlie visual perception (see, e.g. Frisby, 1979). Each analyser reacts to some particular aspect of stimulus input (e.g. black–white, horizontal–vertical or more complicated features). Sutherland supposes that the output of any such analyser can be attached to any response by conditioning. A critical assumption of the theory is that not all analysers are used simultaneously and that it is only when an analyser is being used that its output can determine the response generated. There are, then, two separate processes underlying discrimination learning: learning to use the appropriate analyser (i.e. learning to keep particular analysers switched in or out); and learning which response to attach to the output of this analyser.

Sutherland's theory makes a number of correct, and highly specific, predictions about attentional changes in animals which have been partially reinforced (Note 7.3). However, it does not account for motivational features of reward omission (Section 7.4) nor can it easily handle the way in which different types of schedule result in different amounts of resistance to extinction (see below). There is also at least one instance where its specific predictions do not seem to be fulfilled. McFarland & McGonigle (1967) found that groups of animals trained with either one or two stimulus dimensions available during acquisition showed identical PREEs. The two-dimension group should have had twice as many analysers to switch out and hence should have shown twice as large a PREE. This does not present a great problem for Sutherland's theory of discrimination overall. However, it does negate the specific rule which allowed the theory to predict the occurrence of a PREE and we need not consider the theory further in this chapter. Let us, then, move on to an alternative associative account of the PREE.

Capaldi provides us with an associative account of the PREE which has a somewhat different flavour from Sutherland's. Capaldi (e.g.1967) presumes that each delivery of reward (R) or non-reward (N) produces a specific stimulus after-effect or memory. These traces can become associated with reward during acquisition. Note that (in contrast to Amsel's view – Section 7.4, 7.5) a non-reward is presumed to be a salient event for the animal whether or not there have been previously rewarded trials. Capaldi treats 'non-occurrence of reward' and 'reward omission' as the same event. Further critical assumptions are: that the stimuli of R and N lie on a continuum (from R, through small numbers of N trials to many N trials); that the traces are presumed to remain until they are replaced by other aftereffects; and that the resistance to extinction associated with any stimulus reaches an asymptote with sufficient training.

The main work of the theory is done by the concept of stimulus generalisation. Let us suppose that we train an animal to press a lever whenever a 1000 Hz tone is presented. We can then test it with presentations of other tones of differing frequencies interspersed among the presentations of the 1000 Hz tone. Under these circumstances animals respond maximally to the tone on which they were trained and show progressively less responding as the test tone departs from the original tone. The responding to the test tones is termed generalisation and the fall off in responding with movement of the test tone along the stimulus dimension is termed stimulus generalisation decrement (see Chapter 9 of Mackintosh, 1974, for a review of generalisation).

Let us compare now a group of rats who receive a sequence of trials such as RRRRRRRRRR with a group which receive the sequence NRNRNRNRNR. We assume that both have received enough training for resistance to extinction associated with specific traces to have reached asymptote. What happens when we put them into extinction, i.e. they receive NNNNNNNNNN? The continuously reinforced group will continue to run for a while because the habit strength accrued to the R stimulus will generalise along the R–N continuum to N, NN, NNN etc. However, since generalisation decrement tends to be fairly steep we can assume that they will not run for very long (for example, they might well stop responding after experiencing NNNNNN, see Figure 7.1). The partially reinforced animals, by contrast, have received a number of trials in which running in the presence of the aftereffect of N is reinforced. We have assumed that sufficient trials were given to produce asymptotic resistance to extinction and so they will have the same amount of resistance associated with N as the other group had with R. Thus there will be no decrement in responding

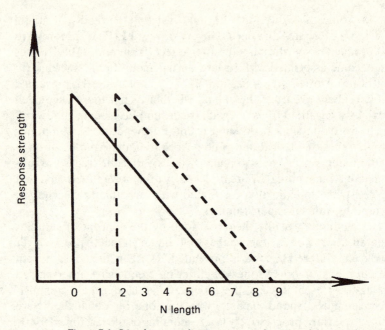

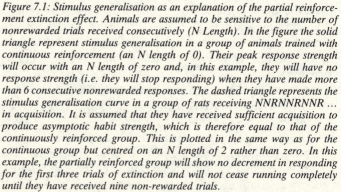

Figure 7.1: Stimulus generalisation as an explanation of the partial reinforce-ment extinction effect. Animals are assumed to be sensitive to the number of nonrewarded trials received consecutively (N Length). In the figure the solid triangle represent stimulus generalisation in a group of animals trained with continuous reinforcement (an N length of 0). Their peak response strength will occur with an N length of zero and, in this example, they will have no response strength (i.e. they will stop responding) when they have made more than 6 consecutive nonrewarded responses. The dashed triangle represents the stimulus generalisation curve in a group of rats receiving NNRNNRNNR ... in acquisition. It is assumed that they have received sufficient acquisition to produce asymptotic habit strength, which is therefore equal to that of the continuously reinforced group. This is plotted in the same way as for the continuous group but centred on an N length of 2 rather than zero. In this example, the partially reinforced group will show no decrement in responding for the first three trials of extinction and will not cease running completely until they have received nine non-rewarded trials.

on the first trial of extinction (N) because no generalisation is required. Thereafter, as the extinction sequence becomes more and more discri-minable from the sequence of N trials which was rewarded during acquisition, decrement will gradually develop. This will, of course, happen more slowly than for the continuously reinforced group of animals. Hence we will see a PREE (Note 7.4).

7.7. Attention, aftereffects, toughening up and frustration

The four theories we have been considering are not incompatible with each other.

Our analysis of Sutherland's theory suggests that it accounts well for changes in selective attention which result from reward omission but that it does not account for the persistent responding demonstrated in the PREE. We can therefore accept a modified version of his theory but need additional accounts of the PREE itself.

Capaldi makes an excellent case for the importance of sequential patterns of after-effects in the control of extinction. But this does not rule out stimuli of frustration as part of the stimulus complex, nor does it rule out more general effects of exposure to frustration.

In support of Amsel there is good evidence for the existence of conditioned and unconditioned states of frustration. However, the existence of such states and of stimuli resulting from them in no way precludes a role for other types of stimuli (in the crudest case Capaldi's after-effects could be, for example, crumbs in the whiskers, or the lack thereof).

The toughening up account cannot handle the data on sequential patterns of reward and non-reward. However, we could suppose that frustration can produce both toughening up and stimuli; and that both toughening up and anticipatory frustration could contribute to the PREE when this is not the result of after-effects.

So, in principle, the PREE could be due to a variety of simple associative and emotional processes operating concurrently. Parsimony requires us to ask whether more than one of toughening up, frustrative stimuli and after-effects is in fact operative, and, if so, what conditions determine which will be the more important.

7.8. Behavioural separation of after-effects, stimuli of frustration and toughening up

Capaldi's theory is based on the differing effects which different sequences of reward and non-reward have on extinction. These effects are clear cut and no other theory can account for them. However, they do not always occur. The effects of inter-trial interval (ITI) on the PREE are reviewed by Mackintosh (1974, pp.457–61). Long intertrial intervals result in a reduced PREE and, more importantly for our present argument, they also eliminate the sequential effects on which Capaldi's theory is based. 'Perhaps the most generally accepted suggestion is that resistance to extinction is mediated by conditioned frustration at long ITIs, and both by conditioned frustration and by the after-effects or traces of preceding outcomes at short ITIs.' (Mackintosh, 1974, p.458).

The transfer of control between after-effects and stimuli of frustration could result from a change in relative salience of particular classes of stimuli. Let us suppose that both after-effects and frustrative stimuli are available to the animal under most conditions. At short intertrial intervals (and with small numbers of trials) specific sequences of rewarded and non-rewarded trials may be relatively easy to remember, hence after-effects will largely control responding. With longer intervals and greater numbers of trials the internal stimuli of conditioned frustration are likely to be more salient predictors of the forthcoming events.

In addition to intertrial interval, the section of the straight alley appears to be an important determinant of the processes operating (see e.g. Godbout, Ziff & Capaldi, 1968; Ziff & Capaldi, 1971). Most experiments divide a straight alley into start, run and goal sections and measure running speed separately in each section. Chen & Amsel (1977) found toughening up only in the start section of their alley, a result which is consistent with indirect evidence from other experiments (Brown & Wagner, 1964, see below). If toughening up determines some part of the PREE, this must be restricted to the start section of the alley.

7.9.   Pharmacological separation of after-effects, stimuli of frustration and toughening up

The behavioural evidence suggests that the PREE can result from all three of the processes we have been considering. More convincing evidence for a separation of processes is provided by experiments which have investigated the effects of anxiolytic drugs (minor tranquillisers) on the PREE. In this context it should be noted that 'anxiolytic' drugs do not block unconditioned frustration as measured in the Amsel-Roussel double runway paradigm (Ison, Daly & Glass, 1967; Gray & Dudderidge, 1971); their action is rather on conditioned frustration as measured by inhibition of responding in anticipation of reward omission (Ison, Daly & Glass, 1967). This parallels the variations in hormonal reactions discussed in the previous chapter.

Anxiolytics do not affect the PREE if acquisition is carried out with a short intertrial interval (Ziff & Capaldi, 1971); but can virtually eliminate the PREE in the goal section of an alley when a 24-hour intertrial interval is used (Feldon, Guillamon, Gray, De Wit & McNaughton,

1979). The simplest explanation of this effect is that anxiolytic drugs interact with conditioned frustration in some way and that the PREE in the goal depends on conditioned frustration only at long intertrial intervals and depends on after-effects of non-reward at short intertrial intervals. (As we noted above, the goal PREE does not depend on toughening up at all.)

The PREE has been investigated with moderate rewards, and relatively short intertrial intervals. Under these conditions anxiolytics have little effect if they are given during both acquisition and extinction. However, the PREE is reduced by a change in drug state, either from drug to saline or saline to drug (Ison & Pennes, 1969). This state dependency (Overton, 1966) is clearly separate from the direct action of the drug seen with a 24-hour intertrial interval in the goal section of the alley.

State-dependent drug effects on the PREE are seen in the start section of the alley even when a 24-hour intertrial interval is used (Feldon *et al.*, 1979). Symmetrical state-dependency, that is to say a reduction in the PREE which is equal in size for both drug–saline and saline–drug shifts, can be accounted for by a contamination with stimulus effects of the drugs of the after-effects of non-reward (Note 7.5).

However, in contrast to a modest reduction in the PREE produced by saline–drug transfer, Feldon *et al.* (1979) found an abolition of the PREE in animals receiving drug in acquisition and saline in extinction. We can attribute *part* of the effect in the drug–saline group to interaction of the drug state with stimulus after-effects of the same type as accounts for the effects in the saline–drug group. But if this were the sole cause of the drug effect saline–drug and drug–saline effects should be equal (Note 7.5). To what can we attribute the remainder of the drug effect? An interaction with frustration is one possibility – but this does not explain why such an interaction should be different in the goal section.

An interaction with toughening up is more likely since this appears restricted to the start section (Chen & Amsel, 1977). If anxiolytics reduce the *aversiveness* of reward omission, we can explain the observed results in the following manner. In the drug–drug and saline–saline groups the aversiveness of non-reward will be the same in acquisition and in extinction. The amount of toughening up in acquisition will, therefore, be sufficient in each case to counteract the unpleasantness of extinction. However, with drug in acquisition and saline in extinction only a small amount of toughening up will occur and this will be followed by a large amount of aversiveness in extinction and hence little resistance. We can, then, attribute the asymmetric nature of the observed state-dependency to a reduction produced by the drug–saline shift in non-associative toughening up (Note 7.6).

In the start section of the alley, then, we have evidence for two components to the PREE when a 24-hour intertrial interval is used. One can be blocked by a drug–saline state change but not by saline–drug, and is likely to be the result of non-associative toughening up. The second is blocked by symmetric changes in drug state and is probably based on stimulus after-effects compounding with the stimulus properties of the drug state.

The PREE appears to depend on each of stimulus after-effects, stimuli of frustration and toughening up with the variables of intertrial interval and alley section interacting to determine the extent to which any particular process contributes to it (Note 7.7).

7.10.   The teleonomy of feelings

In the first part of this chapter I presented arguments for the general functionality of the PREE. An optimal foraging analysis showed that persistence in the face of partial reinforcement is a generally appropriate strategy. (More detailed analysis could well uncover specific environmental situations where this rule would not be optimal – however, for the present argument, these cases would be unimportant provided they would occur only rarely under the conditions in which the animal under consideration evolved.)

When an animal behaves in what (according to optimal foraging theory) is an optimal manner there is no reason to suppose, as Krebs *et al.* (1983) noted, that it is solving the same kind of equations as the theorist. More likely is a gradual accretion of rules of thumb, each of which will produce optimality in a limited range of circumstances. The phylogenetic ubiquity of the PREE and the broad range of circumstances under which any individual species shows the PREE would then be accounted for by the general optimality of persistence as shown by theory – while we would expect that the mechanism of the PREE could vary widely from species to species and from occasion to occasion within a species.

In the case of the rat in the runway, we have experimental evidence for what appear to be at least three separate rules of thumb (after-effects, toughening up, stimuli of anticipatory frustration) which are used to generate persistence.

Given the presence of normal mechanisms of conditioning and

generalisation it is not difficult to see how the control of persistence in extinction by after-effects could have been selected for. All that is necessary is that a non-reward (even with no previous history of reward) should be a salient circumstance for the animal – and this might not require any special selection pressure from the partial rein-forcement situation, it might be a simple consequence of the animal's other perceptual processes. Given the detection by the animal of a stimulus dimension such as N-length, coupled with the phenomenon of stimulus generalisation decrement, which occurs in all major sensory modalities, we would expect a PREE to occur. Subsequently, the utility of the PREE would prevent any tendency for such persistence to be selected against.

In the case of frustration we can construct a similar teleonomic argument to that which we have discussed previously for the evolution of expressions. The basic premise of this argument is that the role of frustration in the PREE represents the development of a secondary function, superimposed on the original function for which frustration evolved. We assume that anticipatory frustration evolved the capacity to produce physiological change initially in response to purely phy-siological (Cannon-type) pressure. It is certainly clear that anticipa-tory frustration does produce changes in peripheral physiological state (see Chapter 5). We can assume that such changes would be clearly perceptible to the animal, and would be likely to bring behaviour under interoceptive control (Slucki *et al.*, 1965). Even if this were not so initially, selection or mutation would have resulted in it becoming so. Internal stimuli associated specifically with anticipatory frustration would then become part of the stimulus complex controlling persist-ence in extinction. The specific selection pressure we invoke for this is the greater range of situations (particularly in the case of long inter-trial intervals) over which the frustration based persistence allows the animal to behave optimally in comparison with those over which the after-effects or other mechanisms are operative.

A similar argument could apply in the case of toughening up. We assume first that anticipatory frustration produces a peripheral phy-siological change for a reason unrelated to the PREE. However, unlike the changes which form the basis of the stimuli of anticipatory frustration discussed in the previous paragraph we assume that the physiological change is not specific to anticipatory frustration, but also occurs in response to anticipatory fear. A specific example which would fit this scenario is the release of corticosterone which occurs in response to both anticipatory frustration and anticipatory fear, but does not occur in response to primary frustration and primary fear

(Chapter 5). If we can assume that the physiological change involved would normally have produced response inhibition, then we could account for toughening up simply in terms of adaptation to or habituation to the effects of the hormone or neurotransmitter controlling the change (there are many examples of drugs which have reduced effects with repeated application). Insufficient is known about the mechanisms of toughening up to carry such arguments very far. However, it is clear that a PREE based on toughening up could have evolved because of the wider range of situations over which it would have permitted persistence to occur.

In my opinion none of the above suggestions are particularly contentious. What has to be borne in mind, and what has provided the material for this chapter, is the necessity for determining what is in principle optimal behaviour, since this may not be obvious, and the necessity for determining some at least of the basic control mechanisms of observed behaviour, before a teleonomic argument can be constructed. In the present case both the optimality analysis and the mechanistic analysis on which the teleonomic argument is based are complicated and need further confirmation. Nonetheless, the general form of the argument shows that stimulus properties of emotions could have functional value and need not be mere epiphenomena. As such the role suggested for them in the previous chapters is not unreasonable, although the specific teleonomy of particular feelings in each particular emotion remains to be assessed. It is clearly possible that some emotional feelings need have no contribution to the control of the relevant emotion – lacking any selection pressure of the type invoked here for the PREE – while nonetheless contributing to the sensory experience of that emotion in the animal experiencing it.

8:   Do emotions mature or differentiate?

Train up a child in the way that he should go:

and when he is old, he will not depart from it.

Proverbs, XXII, 6

8.1.   Teleonomy and procreation

In the previous chapters we have treated emotions as if their exact form were fixed genetically and only minor variations would occur as a result of differing experience in different individuals. We have also considered emotions for which teleonomy can be largely assessed in terms of the survival of the individual (which is then taken to imply an increased probability of reproductive success). The present chapter departs from both of these approaches. While individual survival is necessary it is not sufficient for positive selection pressure. As has been argued in a particularly elegant form by Dawkins (1978), what is really critical is the survival of the genes which code for any particular phylogenetic characteristic. Such survival is highly dependent in higher organisms on successful parent–infant interactions.

The major emotion associated with such interactions in most people's minds would be love (Note 8.1). However, in addition to this there must be an important contribution to the infant's well-being from the fact that parents will be the main, and usually sole, source of virtually all of its homeostatic needs. We might presume from this that the neonate would be supplied with a variety of innate responses which would tend to elicit appropriate behaviour or sustenance from the parents. Equally, it would clearly be advantageous if the neonate could adjust its responses to match parentally determined contingencies. The question arises, then, as to how far there are specific innate systems in the infant and how far the neonate's behaviour is shaped by the parents. In looking at this question we will find that developmental, and particularly comparative developmental, data can give us extensive information about the diversity and structure of emotions which is not easy to obtain from simple studies of adult animals. The developmental course taken by emotions, and the disruption of that course, tends to suggest specific answers to questions such as whether there are in fact different control systems for different emotions, and to what extent different components of a specific adult emotion are controlled by identical systems.

8.2.   Emotional development and emotional maturation

The emotional behaviour of young animals is different from that of adults in that it is frequently more extreme and can occur in different contexts from the adult. In part, this is due to the acquisition of information about the world, e.g. learning which particular things to react to. In part, it can be due to poorly developed motor systems. Largely, I will argue, it is because the emotional systems themselves are not fully functional in the young. The question that arises, then, is whether apparently separate adult emotional systems are the result of experience or the result of maturation.

Consider ordinary motor behaviour. If a new born infant is held so that its legs just touch the ground it will make walking motions. Many months are required, however, before the muscles and joints mature to the point where this in-built motor program can be used properly. By contrast to the maturation of walking, there is no evidence to suggest that bicycle riding is not entirely learned. We have at least two possibilities – emotions might develop through learning, differentiating some single primitive source of emotion. Alternatively, emotions might simply mature at varying rates with no capacity for the environment to influence the adult result.

One of the early proponents of the 'differentiation' position is Bridges (1931). She carried out a large observational study on children and concluded that the first emotions to be differentiated in infancy are distress at shock and interference, and delight in response to satisfying stimuli. According to Bridges, during the pre-school period, fear, anger, joy and affection are recognisable, as well as the earlier evolved excitement, distress and delight. Other emotions such as shame, disgust, anxiety (to be differentiated from e.g. separation distress), revenge, disappointment, jealousy, envy, hope, elation, parental and sexual affection become differentiated or develop later. The way in which emotional behaviour appears to develop in humans, therefore, suggests ever finer differentiation of primary distress and delight. Such observations are not, of themselves, inconsistent with a maturational view – but they would not necessarily have been predicted by it. Equally, by analogy with motor maturation, the fact that certain emotions can be 'recognised' progressively during development does not guarantee that the emotional control system itself is not present from birth and that clear expression of the emotion is what is progressive.

8.3. Do innate emotional expressions imply innate emotions?

By contrast to the suggestion that emotions differentiate, Chapter 4 made the case that emotional *expressions* have a large innate component. Consistent with this, Izard & Buechler (1979), for example, have argued that 'emotion expressions emerge ontogenetically as they become adaptive in the life of the infant and particularly in infant-caregiver communications and relationships'. Thus the apparent differentiation of expressions is attributed not to a process such as learning but simply to the maturation of specific portions of the nervous system. This suggestion is supported by the very tight schedule of appearance of specific expressive behaviours linked to the appropriate context observed across a range of studies. Thus, signs of interest, what is termed the 'endogenous' smile and startle are all present at birth; disgust and distress occur between 0–3 months; the 'social' smile at 1.5–3 months; laughter at 4–5 months; anger at 3–7 months; and fear at 5–9 months (although Darwin reports expressions of fear at 0–5 months). Both the order and time of appearance of these expressions seems too rigid to be due to simple differentiation through experience. Such innateness of expression and differential maturation of differing expressions argues for a similar innateness and differential maturational sequence of the underlying emotions. (There need not be a tight connection between the maturation of expression and the maturation of the equivalent emotion and I will argue below that emotions can be well differentiated even when expression is still undifferentiated.)

In some respects this is not entirely conclusive. For example, Brannigan & Humphries (1972) in an ethological analysis of children's expression identified 70 separate facial units of expression and while 'many facial units ... can be seen during the first day after birth ... there is no evidence to refute the possibility that units of expression are maintained, partly shaped and assigned to specific context in the behavioural repertoire by operant learning'. In particular, the link between specific expressions and specific emotions need not be innate. Expressions could be incorporated, through learning, into emotional systems as these differentiate. This seems especially possible since behavioural patterns in young animals frequently occur entirely outside the motivational context in which they appear in adulthood

(Hinde, 1966). For example, the great tit when young pecks at small objects on the ground only when *not* hungry – when hungry, it begs for food from its parents. Similarly, puppies fed from a bottle with a large hole in it will suck more when the bottle is empty than when it is full – the sucking is not motivated entirely, or perhaps at all, by hunger.

It may be, then, that while expressions are largely innate they become attached through learning to emotions which are themselves the result of differentiation of some primary emotion by experience. The observed linkage between expression and a particular emotion would be ascribed to the fact that most members of a particular species will have a similar early conditioning history. (A failure to attach feeding behaviour to appropriate motivational systems may underlie a range of sometimes paradoxical features of the behaviour of obese humans. Such people tend to eat large amounts of food only when it is palatable, they find it relatively easy to fast, and they can easily adapt their eating patterns to changes of time zone. It appears that, unlike non-obese people whose food intake can be controlled by internal calorie requirements, obese people control their food intake through the use of external cues – Schachter, 1971.) The developmental sequence, therefore, cannot be taken as hard evidence for or against the existence in the neonate of a number of genetically separate emotions. The same is not the case with manipulations which interfere with the normal developmental environment.

8.4.   Immediate effects of separation from parents

The interactions between the mother as care-giver and the developing infant are not purely quantitative. Analysis of the effects of separation of the infant from the mother reveal effects which are not only complex in the dialectical sense (see Chapter 10) but also provide evidence for a selective effect of different components of the mother's behaviour on different specific aspects of the child's behaviour when adult.

In a variety of species absence of the mother results in a period of agitation followed by a period of depression in the infant. These two features of separation distress do not result, however, from the operation of a single controlling factor. While agitation is a common initial response to removal of the mother, the extent to which depression is observed depends on the type of social structure of the groups involved. For example, bonnet macaques differ from pigtail macaques in tending to cluster in groups. When the mother of an infant is removed from each of these types of monkey very different effects occur. In the pigtail monkeys, which tend to live in groups of only a few individuals, the infant shows an extreme reduction in motor activity, a facial expression which can only be described as one of grief and generally shows severe depression. A bonnet infant, by contrast, shows no such reaction, but shows an increased interaction with other bonnet adults which results in solicitous behaviour on their part, and in some cases adoption.

The adaptive value of these patterns of behaviour has been noted by a number of authors. In particular Kaufman & Rosenblum (1969) who obtained the above data note that 'the agitated stage ... would ordinarily succeed in effecting reunion with the mother. The depressed stage, with marked curtailment of movement, the rolled up body with oft-hidden face and the general reduction of interaction with others, would appear to conserve energy and to reduce the likelihood of attack, i.e. to sustain and prolong life until relief might be obtained. [Further] our studies support [the] view that the emotional aspects of the two stage response we saw, both phenomenologically and in their communicated effect upon human observers, did indeed appear to be related to anxiety and depression [respectively]'.

Such distinctive and adaptive behaviour implies the presence of at least one specific emotional system in the neonate. Can separate emotional systems be discerned in the absence of such distinctive reactions?

8.5.   Distinct emotional reactions in the neonate

Scott (1980) has attempted to assess the separateness of emotional systems in the neonate by investigating interactions between stimuli in very young animals. The argument runs as follows. If different stimuli all activate a primal emotional system then interactions between such stimuli will be additive. Any deviation from such additivity is therefore evidence for the presence of separate systems – even when the observed responses to the stimuli do not differ qualitatively, or when the responses differ from those we would expect in an adult. Scott's experimental situation was based on the fact that from about 3 weeks of age puppies show extensive vocalisation if they are separated from their mothers, or if hungry, or if startled by a loud noise. These could all be examples of a single primary state of distress (cf. Bridges, 1931). How stimulus specific are they and how do they interact?

Stimulus specificity is most easily demonstrated with separation from the mother. Separation distress results in as many as 100 yelps per minute continuing indefinitely, thus providing a stable baseline for later measurements. Giving the puppy food or novel objects has no effect on this vocalisation. Contact with soft objects or an unfamiliar puppy produces some reduction. Contact with a familiar puppy produces a large reduction. If the experimenter plays with the puppy this has the greatest effect. This shows both stimulus specificity and interpretation of a fairly high order. Note, for example, that a familiar puppy is very much more effective than a strange puppy – showing that the physical properties of the stimulus are not the critical feature. Likewise gentling by the experimenter, who was not, to my knowledge, perceptibly canine, was highly effective. Mere specificity of eliciting stimulus, however, does not imply that the distress elicited was different from that which could be elicited by other means.

Scott carried out a variety of interaction tests. For example, separation of the puppy from its mother at feeding time blocked eating and produced the same amount of vocalisation as separation at other times. Thus separation distress appeared to block hunger and hunger did not affect separation distress. That this is not due to a ceiling level of vocalisation is shown by a second interaction. Cooling a puppy can produce vocalisation and the combination of isolation and cooling produces more vocalisation than either alone. Thus hypothermia and separation distress are additive. Finally, a sudden loud noise can produce considerable vocalisation – and the amount produced is independent of whether the puppy is isolated or not. Thus, startle is independent of separation distress.

These results provide good evidence for the presence of more than one innate control system underlying behavioural signs of distress – despite the fact that the behavioural signs are not themselves well differentiated in the young. Different classes of environmental stimuli produced non-additive changes in observed behaviour. A further question is: how far was any one of these complex stimuli itself eliciting a unitary reaction?

Hofer (1972) carried out experiments in which he measured the responses of young rats to removal from their mother. In contrast to Scott, he measured an internal response, heart rate, as well as observing the animal's behaviour. His question was: 'Is the young rat responding to all aspects of the experience taken together as a form of gestalt or complex patterned stimulus? If this were the case, omission of one or two components would alter the pattern ... Alternatively, the individual components of the experience could be additive ... [or] the response to separation might depend primarily on one aspect ... the other components being incidental'. Harlow's experiments, discussed in Section 8.8 suggest that the first of these possibilities is not the case.

He found that replacement of some of the components of social interaction normally provided by the mother can compensate to a large extent for her removal. The same conclusion can be drawn from the effectiveness of handling by the experimenter in reducing vocalisation in Scott's experiments.

Hofer removed rats from their mothers at 2 weeks of age and measured heart rate of the removed rat relative to an unremoved litter mate. He found that removal lowers heart rate. This result was not due to a reduction in the temperature of the infant, nor to loss of food *per se* since the removed rat was bottle fed every four hours. He found that frequent feeding with milk (but not a non-nutrient solution) did result in a return of heart rate to normal. He concluded that 'heart rate of the normally mothered rat pups of this age may be maintained at high levels by provision of milk by the mother'.

He also tested the rats behaviourally, by placing them in an unfamiliar box four at a time. Compared with rats which had only just been removed from their mothers, rats which had been isolated for 18 hours showed increases in locomotion, grooming, defecation and urination. Initially, presentation of nutrient *and* non-nutrient solutions eliminated the behaviours, but this was not so after 1 hour of testing. This pattern is totally unlike that seen with the cardiac response. Further, the presence of a non-lactating foster mother blocked the separation response for most of the behaviours measured. 'Thus ... the behavioural effects of maternal separation ... are not mediated by a nutritional mechanism as are the cardiac rate changes, but depend on some aspect of the behavioural interactions between mother and pup'.

Harlow & Harlow (1962) performed a much quoted series of experiments on manipulation of the comfort-attachment stage of development in monkeys. An initial interesting finding relates to the relative importance of furryness as opposed to food for the young monkey. The result is perhaps most crucial for those who would like to account for the development of attachment to a mother in terms of conditioning through food reinforcement. Harlow & Harlow separated young monkeys from their natural mothers and supplied them with two types of somewhat monkey-shaped surrogate: one made of wire and one made of cloth. Feeding bottles could be presented via either type of surrogate. They found that the young monkeys spent approximately 18 hours per day on the cloth surrogate and 1 hour per day on the wire one, independently of which one provided food.

Some of the monkeys were raised with both wire and cloth surrogates and some only with wire ones. This led to further interesting results. 'The development of a security stage was first brought to our attention during a test of fear in the home cage. A mechanical bear or mechanical dog was presented suddenly by raising an opaque screen and exhibiting one of the monsters in an adjacent chamber. After 20 days of age, the infants raised with both cloth and wire surrogates usually fled from the monster and clung intimately to the cloth mother ... this led the infants to relax quickly ... . In the presence of the [surrogate] mother, the behaviour of the infants raised with single wire mothers was both quantitatively and qualitatively different from that of infants raised with cloth mothers. Not only did most of these infants spend little or no time touching their mother surrogates, but the presence of the mother did not reduce their emotionality' (Harlow & Harlow, 1962).

Overall, the observations with wire and cloth 'mothers' provide us with good evidence for two different sources of sustenance provided by the natural mother to an infant – with different contributions to subsequent emotional behaviour. As we might expect even the cloth surrogate, while providing some degree of security, is far from substituting for the interactive attentions of a natural mother. This is brought out by observations on the subsequent development of surrogate-raised monkeys (Section 8.7).

Equally, Hofer's data provide us with evidence that different internal components of what we might like to think of as the same emotion are under the control of these different sources of sustenance – although in the animal's natural environment it has to be admitted that the different stimuli involved would all originate from the same object! Given this complexity of neonatal reactions, is there a role for developmental, rather than maturational, changes in the determination of the adult form of emotional systems?

8.6.   The effects of perinatal manipulations on adult behaviour

The most widely used procedure for manipulating rats in infancy has been handling. The pups are removed from the home cage ... placed in some sort of container ... where they remain for a brief period of time ... and then returned to the home cage. This procedure is usually administered once a day. The number of days of handling [varies]. The relation between handling in infancy and later emotionality has been well established: handled animals are less emotional than nondisturbed controls, and these differences may last for almost the whole of the animal's lifetime. This phenomenon has been documented [using] the open field; activity and defecation measures in an avoidance learning situation; consummatory behaviour; a measure of timidity when emerging from the home cage; and ratings of emotionality.

(Denenberg, 1967)

Handling has also been found to affect hormonal release in a manner consistent with these changes in behaviour (e.g. Levine, Halt-meyer, Karas & Denenberg, 1967). Shock delivered in infancy has the same behavioural effects as handling unless the intensity of shock is particularly high.

It is clear, then, that the emotionality of the rats is modifiable during development. The equivalent of handling, in the normal environment, would be provided by the mother and this allows for both her personality and her environmental experience to affect her offspring. Each does so, with surprisingly similar effects.

Handling of the mother during pregnancy reduces the subsequent emotionality of her offspring. Likewise handling of the mother during her infancy (which reduces her emotionality) also reduces her offspring's emotionality. Equally, shocking the mother during pregnancy increases the emotionality of her offspring.

Denenberg (1967) concludes that 'when two such divergent techniques as shocking mothers during the nursing period and classifying nonpregnant females on the individual difference measures of open field activity yield similar results with respect to their offspring's emotional behaviour, one has considerable confidence that the phenomenon has some degree of generality'. He also cites circumstantial evidence for similar results in human beings: tactile stimulation of infants in institutions is reported to reduce the decline in developmental quotients usually seen. This suggests that the usual decline is due to loss of such stimulation. He also cites evidence that societies which apply mild physical stress to infants show (as in animals) increases in adult height of 2–3 inches. (This does not mean that all men over 6 feet have been circumcised!)

Studies of longer-term effects of maternal deprivation have also provided evidence for the separate nature of emotional systems.

8.7. Long-term effects of early environment on adult behaviour

In Section 8.5 we noted that food and furryness are separate aspects of the mother from the point of view of a young monkey and that it is furryness that leads to attachment and security. Harlow & Harlow (1962) found that despite the effectiveness of the cloth surrogate in reducing emotionality, infants raised on them showed abnormal development at ages ranging from 3–5 years. In fact, by this stage their social responses, heterosexual responses and mothering responses were all as badly affected as those of infants raised in a simple wire cage with no surrogates at all. Harlow & Harlow analysed the contribution to these deficiencies of various components of the normal experience denied these monkeys. An isolated monkey lacks not only maternal care but also experience of interaction with other monkeys, old and young. If young monkeys, isolated from their mothers, are caged together they show a number of abnormal responses – unusually large amounts of clinging and poor development of play. However, the development of heterosexual and social behaviour are unaffected. By contrast an infant raised by a normal mother, but with no opportunity to play with other infants, shows grossly abnormal sexual and play behaviour, with normal development of social behaviour. A variety of other manipulations show a variety of effects (Table 8.1) which suggest that there is no unitary underlying pathological change which can explain the varying deficiencies in each of play, social reactions and sexual behaviour.

These data suggest that different aspects of early experience contribute to the normal development of different behavioural systems. The fact that experience limited to interaction with other infants can lead to essentially normal defensive and sexual reactions argues strongly that such reactions have a major innate component rather than being largely learned by observation of agonistic and sexual behaviour of adults. Equally, the fact that appropriate rearing conditions can eliminate defensive and sexual reactions argues for an important contribution from experience. We may also conclude, through the same

Table 8.1 *Patterns of play (P), defensive social behaviour (D) and Sexual behaviour (S) after various types of intervention during infancy. Data modified from Harlow & Harlow (1962). Amount of behaviour of the relevant type is graded from 0 (absent) to 4 (normal).*

| | Amount of behaviour observed | | | | |
	0	1	2	3	4
Normal Mother/ play allowed					PDS
No Mother/ 4 infants per cage/ play allowed				P	DS
Surrogate Mother/ play allowed				S	PD
'Motherless' Mother/ play allowed			D	S	P
Normal Mother/ no play	S	P			D
Isolated 80 days			PDS		
Isolated 6 months	DS	P			
Isolated 2 years	PDS				

logic as was used in relation to Scott's data, that the differential pattern of disturbance of reactions with differing rearing conditions argues strongly for the presence of separate underlying systems – although the data could be handled by a carefully formulated 'differentiation' position. (However it is difficult to see why infants caged together, with plenty of opportunity for play, show normal defensive and sexual behaviour but retarded development of play.)

8.8. Do emotions mature and differentiate?

Harlow & Stagner (1933) suggested that 'unconditioned affective responses form a basis for the emotions ... . Emotions themselves are conditioned responses subsequently formed. The conditioning processes, by which all emotions are acquired, modify the unconditioned affective pattern by enormously extending the range of stimuli which will elicit it, and usually by damping the violence of the unconditioned affective response'. Thus the data so far suggest that, in considering emotions, we must take into account the presence of some number of different, primary, innate, releasing systems; and that each such system can be modified by experience. Where such modification is an expansion of the potential eliciting stimuli there is also the possibility that some stimuli could simultaneously elicit reactions via more than one primary system to produce a complex result.

Harlow's monkey experiments showed differential effects of different aspects of isolation on the development of different skeletal responses. Hofer's results strongly imply not only that autonomic responses are also subject to differential developmental pressures but also that these pressures may be different from those moulding the skeletal system. Thus autonomic responses could well develop somewhat independently of the skeletal responses with which they are normally associated. Indeed, differential development could account for the regularity of within-subject peripheral reactions to specific emotional stimuli coupled with the variability of such reactions from subject to subject (Schnore, 1959). How does such plasticity fit with a view of emotions as dependent on innate releasing systems?

A problem only arises if one wishes to dichotomise innateness and plasticity – this is shown best by analogy with the visual system (see Frisby, 1979). The visual (striate) cortex is normally organised in an apparently standard way so that it is tempting to see this organisation as the result of direct genetic control. However, if young animals are brought up in an unusual visual environment, the organisation of the visual cortex changes. The change is not, however, random – instead it can be described as an increase in the number of analytic units which react to common features of the environment and a decrease in those which analyse uncommon features. So it is clear that, although the organisation of the normal adult visual cortex is under genetic control, the genes produce their results at one remove, via interaction with the visual environment of the young animal. The common organisation of most adult visual cortices is at least in part attributable to a common type of visual environment during development for members of that species.

It seems reasonable to suppose that a similar combination of genetic foundation and developmentally influenced superstructure could exist for emotional systems. Thus, the developmental data show that there are indeed, in the neonate, separate innate systems which form the basis for separate adult emotions. However, they also suggest that the normal form of each adult emotion depends on the appropriate moulding, during development, of a number of innate components. In this context it is particularly noteworthy that what may appear superficially in a neonate to be a complex reaction coordinated by some central organisational process may in fact reflect a number of separate functional units. It is also clearly possible that each basic innate unit (which might be skeletal, autonomic, etc.) could be incorporated into more than one emotion.

9: Cognition, learning and emotion

Pluralitas non est ponenda sine necessitate.

Propose plentiful parameters only when pushed.
Gulielmus de Occam: Quodlibeta, V, Q.i

9.1. What place has learning in the analysis of emotion?

In the initial parts of this book the internal and external expressions of emotions were treated as if they are fixed both in form and in terms of adequate releasing stimuli. However, the previous chapter shows that the exact form of adult emotional reactions depends on early experience – and hence in some sense on learning. Learning is also a critical factor in determining adequate stimuli for many organisms. It will be remembered from Chapter 2 that the adequacy of a stimulus for the release of a state-dependent reflex depended on the interpretation of the stimulus by the animal rather than any gross aspect of the physical characteristics of the stimulus complex.

In this context the study of animal learning is important for two different reasons. First, it gives us a way of studying scientifically (and hence in the terms of the present book biologically) the modifiable aspects of the control of emotional behaviour, which are not amenable to comparative analysis because they differ from individual to individual even within the same species. Second, it provides us with a means of assessing the internal states and processes which give rise to emotional behaviour and the nature of the adequate stimuli which give rise to those states. In this sense learning theory can provide us with an assessment of cognitive factors in animals.

To show that these questions of internal state and process can be addressed objectively, we will review the status of emotion within learning theory.

Learning theory has for many years been a stronghold of radical behaviourism. Few psychologists would ask radical behaviourists to provide us with a concept such as emotion. As Dickinson noted in an earlier volume in this series (1980, p.4) 'According to behaviourism, the job of psychology is to specify the relationship between some physical event in the environment, the stimulus, and, in the case of learning, some acquired behavioural pattern, the response, without reference to mental processes.' Concentration on behavioural observations has led to repeatability and objectivity with respect to experimental data, but at the same time the avoidance of process words in the learning theorists' vocabulary has tended to distance them from other areas of psychology. However, as Dickinson (op.cit. p.5) also points out: 'being limited to observing behavioural changes does not commit you to a [radical] behaviourist perspective. There is no reason why mental processes should not be inferred from behaviour'.

This conclusion is by no means acceptable to all of those who currently study animal learning (Blackman, 1983). Blackman presents a critique of the point of view taken by Dickinson and others. He asks two separate questions. The first is whether the use of a particular cognitive term, i.e. a term which refers back to a particular mental process, by a learning theorist allows, or may be taken to assume, extrapolation from man to rat. The second question is whether it is appropriate to use hypothetical constructs of any type to explain animal behaviour. I will argue below that his negative answer to the first of these questions is correct but that his negative answer to the second is not.

In what follows we will start with arguments which lead to the decision that hypothetical constructs are allowable, provided that suitable behavioural evidence can be obtained for them. This is followed by consideration of specific evidence for specific constructs. The evidence for what are termed two-process theories of learning (see below) is also to a large extent evidence for states which can be given emotion labels and which, therefore, might be seen as emotional states. Emotion labels as used by a learning theorist do not necessarily imply anything more than motivation. The justification in the context of learning theory for reference to emotion except as a synonym for motivation therefore requires further evidence.

Such evidence is provided in the present chapter by consideration of the release of species typical responses. In many cases stimuli used as reinforcers (i.e. rewards and punishments), with the intention on the part of the experimenter of increasing or decreasing the probability of occurrence of a specific response, can result in the generation of complex behaviour patterns, specific to the species being investigated, which are no part of the experimenter's plan. The nature of the patterns observed depends on the presence of adequate releasing stimuli in the animal's environment. Depending on the exact experimental situation such behaviour patterns can enhance or interfere with the response which the experimenter was attempting to manipulate. These behaviour patterns reflect what can be termed emotional as opposed to purely motivational consequences of the states elicited by reinforcing stimuli. An important feature of such species-typical behaviour patterns, and of equivalent effects which require indirect measurement, is that their occurrence is not directly related to the occurrence of the response being reinforced by the experimenter. Typically, such emotional reactions will precede or parallel the reinforced response in the initial stages of learning but will disappear as the reinforced response reaches asymptotic strength.

It seems, then, that behaviour in conditioning experiments provides us with evidence for two types of process: motivational ones, which account for the occurrence and strength of the learned response; and emotional ones, which account for the occurrence and strength of other responses. Our detailed consideration of these conclusions needs to start with the question of how far we are in a position to postulate any internal processes of this type at all.

9.2. Radical behaviourism and cognitive learning theory

According to Blackman the essential difference between cognitive and behavioural analysis is that the latter identifies some functional relationship while the former, in addition, postulates some 'higher process' which does not in fact add explanatory power to the original functional observation. 'Behaviour analysts ... would argue that the increasing complexity of the experimental arrangements which give rise to conditioning may need to be summarised by increasingly sophisticated mathematical or algebraic functions, but such functions clearly summarise the relationships between events rather than possibly represent hypothetical structures within an animal' (Blackman, 1983, p. 43). Dickinson's view is that 'for the cognitive psychologist learning consists of the formation of some novel mental structure which is only indirectly manifest in behaviour, whereas for the behaviourist the development of the new response pattern itself is learning' (Dickinson, 1980, p. 4)

The difference between the two types of approach is exemplified by Dickinson's (1980) and Blackman's (1983) views of the phenomenon of sensory preconditioning.

Sensory preconditioning proceeds as follows. Two stimuli are presented a number of times with one of them preceding, and hence signalling, the occurrence of the other. For example, a tone might be followed by a light. At low intensities neither the stimuli nor their pairing will produce marked changes in behaviour. Next the light is paired with shock. This pairing changes the animal's subsequent responses to the light in a variety of ways. The critical observation is that, despite the fact that the tone is never paired with shock, the animal's responses to the tone are changed in a similar manner; they are 'preconditioned' to the light and this association is then transferred to the shock.

According to Dickinson:

During the first stage, exposure to the tone–light pairings set up some internal representation of this relationship which remained behaviourally silent ... . When the light subsequently acquired significance by being paired with shock, the internal structure representing the tone as a predictor of the light resulted in the tone also becoming fear inducing ... . Since the behaviourist defines learning in terms of a change in behaviour, he would be forced to conclude that little or no learning occurred when the light and tone were paired. Consequently [when we] pair the light with shock, we should not expect to see any change in the behaviour elicited by the tone.   (Dickinson, 1980)

According to Blackman:

Sensory preconditioning can be explained in a similar but more objective way by the behaviour analyst: given that S1 and S2 have occurred in a specified temporal relationship, and that S2 then occurred in a specified relationship with an unconditional stimulus, S1 will elicit a conditioned response when presented alone. Of course this is "just" a restatement of the procedure and its findings. But it ... explains it without recourse to putative events at other, unobservable, levels which may add nothing to the power of the explanation and again might be said to shelter behind some degree of ambiguity.

(Blackman, 1983, p.44).

Many of us would feel that the essence of explanation is specifically that it is not 'just a restatement' of the data, in whatever way restatement is viewed. One of the major uses of scientific theory is extrapolation outside the original experimental domain. In this specific instance, even if we ignore the value of extrapolation, Dickinson's explanation is preferable in another way: surely, he is right when he suggests that the sensory preconditioning experiment allows us to infer that some change has occurred within the animal. Blackman must then be taken as suggesting that we should not theorise about the nature of such changes even when we are sure that they have occurred. But inference about underlying processes has always been a powerful scientific tool. If entities such as electrons and inertia are allowable inferences, why should we not be permitted to infer associations, emotions and the like?

Earlier in his paper Blackman discusses an example of the use of an everyday term as a heuristic device: where the timing behaviour of animals in the absence of external cues is discussed in terms of internal clocks. This mode of speech can lead, by analogy, to questions of whether the clock is running slow, is stopped or has been reset (see Church, 1978). However, Blackman wants no truck with the idea that there is a clock in the rat. If clocks must be mentioned, he would prefer to talk of the rat being the clock. The question is: should we talk about clocks at all?

Two antithetical points should be noted immediately. First, no one would suggest that the animal actually has a metal watch inside itself which it can view in some mysterious way – the notion of a clock must be, at best, analogy. Secondly, there are a number of ways in which an animal can solve a timing problem without using an internal clock, e.g. 'run round the cage three times and then have a wash' could generate a 'timed' interval. So, before we talk about a clock, even as an analogy, we should ensure that our experiments have ruled out other simpler explanations of the apparently 'timed' behaviour.

Provided always that such care is taken, we may well find that concepts such as 'clock' are useful. Let us consider for a moment the diurnal timing of behaviour patterns, rather than the timing studied in animal learning experiments. Not only has the idea of a clock been heuristic in this context, it has also led to the search for, and recent identification of, internal physiological clocks. If the idea of a clock were a mere mathematical abstraction then searching for its physical instantiation would have been a waste of time; and the importance of the suprachiasmatic nucleus, for example, would not have been discovered (see Carlson, 1980, Ch. 15; Zucker, 1983).

However, even Blackman admits that 'the empirical contribution made by cognitive learning theorists to behavioural analysis has been more striking perhaps than that of the behaviour analysts themselves … . Perhaps … cognitive concepts … provide a heuristic device with respect to empirical investigations' (op.cit. p.48). Our discussion of clocks suggests that this heuristic value might arise because the use of cognitive concepts relates directly to actual 'cognitive' processes. To say this is not to suggest, however, that our normal use of cognitive concepts can be transported directly into the study of animal learning.

9.3. Limitations on the valid use of cognitive terms in learning theory

Ritual avoidance of internal if not cognitive concepts has not only limited experimentation in the area of learning theory but, more importantly, has distanced learning theory from other areas of psychology which would have benefited from closer contact. None the less, I fully agree with Blackman on one point: the use of such terms should in no way involve 'extrapolation from humans to animals' (Blackman, 1983). As with the use of a term such as electron, any inferred mental process must rest on its own objective evidential base. I suspect that Dickinson too would agree with this since he explicitly considers the possibility that humans and animals may differ widely in their cognitive structure.

I believe that the use of cognitive terms can best proceed in the opposite direction. Animal species are not identical to man nor are they identical to each other. The general trends which can be seen in evolution give us some hope, however, that the basic forms of behavioural control will be similar in many animals, and that there will be in man analogues of the systems discoverable in other animals. For example, there are many instructive similarities between the digestive systems of cows and men – this does not force us to conclude that humans ruminate or that cows eat meat. The argument has been made elsewhere (Schachter, 1980) that the control of human behaviour may be more biological than self-report of our cognitions suggests; and similarities between emotions in rat and man are specifically considered in Chapter 11. But these similarities do not justify the use of conventional cognitive terms to describe the control processes of animal behaviour. Much of the force of the behaviourist revolution stemmed from its contrast to the unsatisfactory use of introspection and ordinary language terms in psychology.

There is, therefore, one particular aspect of cognitive learning theory which I find unsatisfactory – it uses conventional cognitive terms. I would much prefer that it used totally invented words (e.g. electron). As Blackman points out the use of cognitive words tempts us to go too far beyond the data. However, language contains a range of words which do abstract at least some useful general features of the control of behaviour. It is very hard for the non-specialist, therefore, to see what a psychologist is driving at if these terms are not used. But it does seem to me that Blackman is right when he cautions us against the premature use of cognitive terms. Words like electron and inertia have been coined in the laboratory and their correct use has to be learned within the context of theoretical physics. Words referring to emotions are used in everyday English and come complete with a host of unvoiced assumptions and implications. It is difficult to remember, as we use them, that their meaning must be limited to that provided by experiment and the theories based on such experiments. As I argued in Chapter 1, the everyday assumptions and implications of the words used have probably been the main cause of confusion in the analysis of emotion.

Blackman asks if a cognitive term applied to a rat is intended to imply that the animal shares a particular psychological function with man, including the awareness of that function. 'If this is not the case, it might seem that cognitive terminology may be no more than an attractively daring (and potentially grossly misleading) choice of words to identify hypothetical constructs' (op.cit. p.40). The real danger here, he points out, is that premature use of cognitive terms may 'deflect psychologists away from sound behavioural analyses and the recognition of their explanatory power' (op. cit. p.41).

9.4. The use of emotion words without colloquial implications

The study of emotion has been bedevilled by the indiscriminate use of emotion descriptors, often with different people meaning different things by the same word. Even if we do not go as far as radical behaviourism, we must agree that the unthinking introduction of intervening variables whenever the theoretical going gets rough is to be avoided. However, the emergence of emotion concepts within the vocabulary of learning theorists has occurred against a background of radical behaviourism. Precisely because this is an area where such concepts have been resisted, it is an area where we are likely to find their surest foundation.

However, where a specific motivation or emotion term is derived from the experimental literature, we should be wary of extrapolating directly to any species other than that specifically tested. We should also be prepared to find that, once the psychologist is correctly applying such a term to the human case, its properties and the assumptions which go with it show no obvious parallels with the use of the equivalent word in everyday speech.

9.5. The development of two-process theories of learning

Two-process theories of learning as a class maintain that most learning involves the operation of two independent learning processes (see Rescorla & Solomon, 1967; Mackintosh, 1974; Gray, 1975). Before discussing this theoretical position we should first distinguish the 'two processes' involved at a simpler level – these processes are classical (Pavlovian, respondent, Stimulus–Stimulus, Sign–Significate, S–S) and instrumental (Thorndikian, operant, Stimulus–Response, S–R) conditioning.

At the descriptive level, classical and instrumental conditioning procedures are quite different. In classical conditioning the experimenter arranges a contingency between one stimulus (the conditioned stimulus or CS, e.g. a bell) and another (the unconditioned stimulus or UCS, e.g. a piece of food). After a number of trials when the CS has consistently preceded the UCS the animal will start to respond to the CS (e.g. by salivating). In the classical paradigm there is no programmed relationship between this conditioned response (CR) and the UCS. In instrumental conditioning the experimenter arranges a contingency between a response (e.g. a lever press) and the UCS (e.g. food). A change in the frequency of occurrence of the response is again taken as evidence of conditioning.

There has been considerable controversy as to whether these two distinct types of contingency procedure result in distinct forms of conditioning process. Both the source of controversy and its resolution can be seen in experiments on the autoshaping of responses (Brown & Jenkins, 1968). In autoshaping, a manipulandum (e.g. a key) is illuminated prior to the delivery of food. This is a simple classical conditioning contingency. After a number of pairings of the light and food hungry pigeons will come to peck the manipulandum. Note that once they are doing so they are subject to an instrumental contingency which has not been explicitly programmed since pecking is followed by food. Similarly, it is possible that, before any key pecking occurred, exploratory responses such as moving towards the lit manipulandum were subject to adventitious instrumental reinforcement in a similar manner. Thus, all of the pigeon's responding could be due solely to an instrumental conditioning process. Conversely, it could be argued that in all supposedly instrumental conditioning experiments the unique stimulus configuration presented to the pigeon when it is close to the key (as it must be to peck it) is producing autoshaping through a classical conditioning process.

The contribution of the two separate processes can be assessed by pitting the supposed instrumental and classical contingencies against each other. That is to say we arrange a situation in which the lit key predicts food as before but key-pecking cancels the delivery of the food (an 'omission contingency'). If the operation of the manipulandum is maintained by the classical contingency it should remain at a fairly high level; if, however, it is maintained by the instrumental contingency it should disappear. It turns out that pigeons' responses are largely the result of classical conditioning while rats' responses, at least with respect to the effect of an omission contingency, are under instrumental control (Williams & Williams, 1969; Ridgers & Leslie, 1975 cited by Millenson & Leslie, 1979). It should be noted that the pigeon, despite its continued responding in this situation, is not totally insensitive to the omission contingency. If two keys are available and pecking on one causes omission of reward while pecking on the other is irrelevant, the pigeon will cease pecking on the omission key – but only if the relationship between the lighting of the keys and reward is the same for both keys in all respects other than the omission contingency. (For further discussion of autoshaping see Millenson & Leslie, 1979.)

These and a variety of other experiments (see, e.g. Gray, 1975) support the idea that responding can be changed as a result of both classical and instrumental conditioning contingencies. They also show that in any learning paradigm we must be prepared for the effects of both types of contingency whether explicitly programmed by the experimenter or not.

The next step towards a two-process *theory* is provided by a classical experiment by Miller (1948). He used a box with two compartments – one black and one white. Rats placed into this box showed no preference for a particular compartment before training. He then shocked the rats in one of the compartments. They learned to avoid the shock by running into the second compartment before the shock was switched on. Miller then made two critical changes. No further shocks were delivered; and now the rats could only reach the second compartment if they learned to turn a wheel to open a door between the compartments. A substantial number of the rats learned this new response.

A simple explanation is available for the change in behaviour shown by the rats in the first part of this experiment. Termination of the shock reinforces the connection between the stimuli of the first compartment and the response of running into the second. No internal processes (other than that of reinforcement itself) need be inferred. But what reinforces the wheel-turning response? The most obvious candidate for this is removal of the stimuli of the first compartment. But we know that, initially at least, these stimuli were not punishing for the rats. Miller concluded that fear as a drive became conditioned to the stimuli of the first compartment and that it was termination of this state of fear which reinforced the new response.

Thus, a two-process approach to learning requires that classical conditioning not only produces externally observable responses which can interact with instrumental conditioning, but that it also produces certain classes of internal state.

To take us over this additional hurdle, let us look at an experiment by Solomon & Turner (1962). In their experiment dogs were first trained to press a panel in order to avoid a shock under the control of a visual stimulus. After the response was well learned, the animals were paralysed with curare and received a number of presentations of two tones one of which signalled the occurrence of a shock and the second of which did not. Note that in this phase of the experiment there can be no direct association of the tones with panel pressing since the animal is paralysed and can make no responses. After recovery from the curare the dogs showed avoidance responding controlled by the tone which had signalled shock as well as by the original visual stimulus but not by the tone which had not been associated with shock. Solomon & Turner emphasise that panel pressing was observed as opposed to other forms of behaviour which simple stimulus–shock conditioning might have elicited (e.g. howling, struggling or freezing).

Rescorla & Solomon (1967) say 'this experiment can be analysed in terms of two propositions of two-process learning theory: (a) Pavlovian association processes precede the acquisition of emotional reactions to previously neutral stimuli; and (b) these emotional reactions have motivational properties that can influence instrumental responding'. Solomon & Turner's experiment effectively separates the two components which were merely deduced from the results of Miller's experiment.

Rescorla & Lo Lordo (1965) carried out a series of experiments, in unparalysed animals, which manipulated the classical conditioning component of fear acquisition in a variety of ways. In their first experiment they initially presented a stimulus, CS1, paired with shock. Next a combination of CS1 + CS2 predicted no shock; in their second experiment CS1 predicted shock and CS2 no shock in a discrimination procedure; and in a third experiment CS1 predicted shock when presented alone and predicted no shock if it was preceded by CS2. The effects of these classical training procedures were then assessed by looking at their interaction with previously established shuttle avoidance responding. In all three experiments it was found that CS1 increased the rate of shuttling but that CS2 decreased it. They therefore showed that a number of the procedures described by Pavlov for varying the effects of stimuli in ordinary classical conditioning experiments have similar effects on fear conditioning when this is subsequently assessed by an instrumentally conditioned response.

They carried out one further experiment of interest. There were two separate conditions. In the first a period of no shock during which no stimulus was explicitly presented was followed by a period of no shock with an explicit stimulus (the equivalent of CS2 in the above examples). In the second a period of unsignalled shock was followed by a period of no shock with presentation of CS2. In the second, but not the first, condition CS2 subsequently decreased the rate of shuttle avoidance. Rescorla & Lo Lordo (1965) conclude that 'in order for a stimulus to depress avoidance responding it is sufficient that it previously be explicitly paired with a period free of shock ... against a background in which shock does in fact occur'.

All of the above data are consistent with the idea that classical conditioning can create internal states, and that such states have motivational properties which can interact in an approximately additive manner with other sources of motivation to determine the extent of instrumental responding. Classical conditioning also interacts with instrumental responding, particularly during acquisition, when the classically conditioned reaction is incompatible with the required instrumental response.

9.6. Emotion and the release of species-specific behaviour

We have already discussed one example of incompatibility of classically conditioned and instrumentally conditioned responses – autoshaping with an omission contingency in pigeons. Here the classical pairing of lit key with food elicits a key peck even when the pigeon loses food as a result. An interesting aspect of this behaviour is the nature of the observed response. Pigeons show relatively stereotyped pecking which is different depending on whether food or water is the target. Jenkins & Moore (1973) presented pigeons which were both hungry and thirsty with a key which was lit with a different colour depending on whether food or water was to be delivered. They found that the pigeons effectively 'drank' the key when it signalled water and 'ate' the key when it signalled food. Thus the response, and hence the conditioned internal state, is reinforcer specific.

More importantly the classically conditioned response appears to be a standard part of the animals normal repertoire – a 'species-typical' response. Timberlake & Grant (1975) have argued further that what is conditioned is not just a specific reflex but an 'entire behaviour system' of which the reflex is a part. In their experiment they used a live rat on a platform as the stimulus in an autoshaping experiment with food as the reinforcer. They found that this procedure caused the experimental rats to approach and make social contact with the stimulus rat – they did not attempt to eat the stimulus rat as one might expect on the basis of analogy with the pigeons 'eating' the lit key in the standard autoshaping paradigm. Stimulus rats which were not paired with food were not contacted to the same extent and a rat sized block of wood was not contacted at all. These results are most easily explained by assuming that simple stimulus substitution of a reflex is not occurring, rather the conditioning procedure elicits a change in internal state which can then enable (Chapter 2) particular components of the animal's respondent systems depending on the releasing capacity of the available stimuli – if the stimulus which is paired with food is another rat we see begging rather than eating directed at the stimulus.

This conclusion also follows from a series of experiments carried out by Holland and described by Rescorla (1978). In these experiments a number of behavioural measures (rearing, perambulation, magazine entry, head jerking) were obtained during Pavlovian stimulus–food pairings. The stimulus used was either a light or a high tone. The first finding of interest was that the pattern of acquisition of responding, and the nature of the responses whose occurrence was increased, depended on whether conditioning was to the light or to the high tone. The critical experiment for our purposes involved the use of second-order conditioning. In second-order conditioning a new conditioning stimulus (in Holland's experiment this was a low tone) precedes the previously neutral stimulus (either the light or the high tone) from first-order conditioning in the absence of the original UCS (food). In this second-order conditioning paradigm Holland found that association with the light or the high tone produced highly similar changes in responding to the low tone. Despite that fact, the changes in behaviour to these two stimuli produced by association with food were markedly different. This provides strong evidence that the central states elicited by the light and the high tone in the first-order paradigm are essentially the same and that the difference in behavioural reaction resulting from these central states is determined by the eliciting properties of the stimuli.

Species typical responses can both interfere with, and enhance, responding in a conditioning experiment. With the autoshaping experiments, approach to a stimulus which has been paired with food improves performance since the stimulus is related to the manipulandum. By contrast, Breland & Breland (1961) describe a number of instances in which approach to such a stimulus is incompatible with, and hence impairs the learning of, the rewarded response. The same effects can be seen with punishment. Shock can elicit aggressive behaviour. If aggression is incompatible with the required escape response this will delay conditioning, whereas, if the correct avoidance response is defined by the experimenter as attack, fast conditioning is seen (Azrin, Hutchinson & Hake, 1967). More generally, Bolles (1970) suggested that the great ease with which animals can learn some avoidance responses depends on the existence of species-specific defence reactions (SSDRs) and that 'avoidance learning in the laboratory is possible only if the response we require of our animal is an SSDR or is at least highly compatible with the animal's SSDR repertoire' (Bolles, 1975).

It should be noted, however, that in talking about SSDRs we are not necessarily talking about simple response sequences. Bolles (1975) describes an experiment by Duncan which illustrates this point. Duncan initially tried to train rats to avoid shock by running, in any manner, within a box. The response occurred very frequently, but then actually decreased rather than increased with training. Then a strip of tape was used to separate the floor of the box visually into two parts. The rats now learned the response. One way of describing the rats' behaviour in this experiment would be 'run to a safe place; if there is no safe place then freeze'. Masterson & Crawford (1982) have, in fact, proposed the theory that reinforcement of responding results not from presentation in the case of positive reinforcers and removal in the case of negative ones, but rather from the fact that in both cases the response leads to the animal obtaining positive stimuli. In the case of avoidance the response leads to the animal obtaining a safe place. An experiment by Crawford & Masterson (1978) illustrates this point.

It has often been noted that rats have great difficulty in learning lever press responses to avoid shock. Crawford & Masterson, on the other hand, obtained good learning of lever press avoidance. They argue that the critical feature of the experiment was that lever pressing not only resulted in shock avoidance but also made available a safe compartment. (It may be remembered that in Miller's experiment described at the beginning of this chapter a similar result was obtained.) They found fast acquisition of lever pressing whether the rat was permitted to run from the shock compartment to the safe compartment, or whether lever pressing resulted in the rat being picked up and placed in the safe compartment; and they found the usual poor acquisition of lever pressing when a press resulted in a shock free interval, or when it terminated the stimuli which predicted the shock.

The requirement for compatibility of the to-be-learned response with species-specific reactions can also be demonstrated with appetitive conditioning. For example, Shettleworth (1973) recorded rates of barpressing, digging, scrabbling, open rearing and face washing in hamsters. (Scrabbling involves scraping the paws against a wall while standing up and is different from digging in the way the paws are moved and the body is held; open rearing is rearing in which the paws do not touch walls or floor; see Shettleworth, 1978 for a Table of definitions.) The rates of all but face washing could be increased by food reinforcement. When reinforced for face washing, a hamster would increase the rate of initiation of face washing sessions but would not complete the washing process, rather it 'reared and waved its forepaws a few times on either side of its nose'. This 'lick and a promise' approach must be familiar to anyone who has tried to condition face washing before meals in juvenile *Homo sapiens*.

The selective conditioning of particular responses is not due to intrinsic differences in their conditionability. If shock is used as a reinforcer, the rate of scrabbling is still easily changed, face washing is now changed to some extent and rearing is hardly changed at all (Shettleworth, 1978). It could be argued that the nature of the response is interacting here with the different temporal and other procedural aspects of shock delivery as compared to food delivery. However, a similar pattern of results to those obtained with food delivery was obtained when electrical brain stimulation was used as the positive reinforcer (Shettleworth & Juergensen, 1980).

Data such as the above suggest that a more ecological (Johnston, 1981) approach to the phenomena of learning is warranted. However, great care should be taken in the use of ecological arguments. As Johnston notes, it is very easy, and usually wrong, to provide explanations *ex post facto* in terms of presumed items of an animal's normal repertoire which have contributed to the results of a learning experiment.

9.7.   Emotion as an antidote to motivation

So far we have considered the case where state-dependent reflexes interfere with instrumental responses and, it could be assumed, that both the state-dependent reflexes and the conditioning of the instrumental responses depend on the same underlying internal state. This internal state would normally be identified as motivational – a concept which can have a variety of definitions (Hoyenga & Hoyenga, 1984, Chapter 1) but which in the present context is exemplified by statements of the form 'the food-deprived rat pressing the lever is motivated by hunger'. From the point of view of a radical behaviourist the coexistence of state-dependent reflexes and instrumental responses does not require the postulation of an internal state at all but merely leads to the observation that a particular unconditioned stimulus can reinforce many classes of response and also elicit responses which are incompatible with certain other classes of response which the experimenter may wish to condition. However, two-process accounts of learning offer a deeper kind of incompatibility between classically and instrumentally conditioned reactions.

Estes & Skinner (1941) trained rats to respond for food reinforcement. They then superimposed on the reward contingency presentation of a tone which predicted an unavoidable shock. Neither the tone nor the shock produced any change in responding on the first presentation. After a number of presentations of the tone–shock pairing the responding of the rats was suppressed during the tone. Note that from a reinforcement theorist's point of view this conditioned suppression is surprising. By failing to respond the rat is likely to lose food. Equally, neither responding nor failing to respond affects the delivery of either the shock or the stimulus which predicts the shock. Why does the rat press the lever less? One answer is that fear becomes conditioned to the stimulus and that this fear conflicts with the hunger which is supporting responding.

The conditioned suppression paradigm is sufficiently compelling in this regard to have been called by some 'the conditioned emotional response' (e.g. Millenson & Leslie, 1974). However, before proceeding we should look at some simpler alternative explanations of conditioned suppression: (a) that it involves adventitious punishment of the suppressed response; and (b) that it involves classical conditioning of competing responses.

It is clear that in the conditioned suppression paradigm described above some of the animal's responses will be followed by shock. This represents inadvertant punishment of the response. It is admittedly weak in that many responses will not be followed by shock. However, conditioned suppression is usually weak in relation to response contingent punishment. An answer to this objection is provided by Millenson & De Villiers (1972). They investigated the effect of superimposing a conditioned suppression paradigm on a baseline in which two responses were being made concurrently. They found that the less frequent of the two baseline responses was more suppressed than the more frequent. Since the latter was more closely associated with shock this result contradicts the punishment hypothesis (see Millenson & De Villiers for a discussion of a number of other experiments).

The competing response hypothesis is very similar to the two process hypothesis. The difference is that, instead of a hypothetical internal state, it is presumed that some externally observable response becomes conditioned and competes with the baseline response. Certainly, during conditioned suppression training, animals show a variety of responses (defecation, urination, piloerection, jumping, freezing) some of which could in principle interfere with the baseline. However, if suppression results from conditioning of a response incompatible with lever pressing, say, it should not matter how the lever pressing is reinforced. There are at least two instances in which this is not the case. The simplest to understand is the superimposition of a CS for shock on a response which is itself reinforced with avoidance of shock. In this case the CS produces an increase in responding not a decrease (Waller & Waller, 1963; Weisman & Litner, 1972). The two-process account of this is straightforward. The CS elicits fear. The response is the result of fear. So, responding is increased. The second instance is the superimposition of a CS for shock on a baseline of differential reinforcement for low rates of response (DRL). This is a schedule in which the rat is rewarded for every lever press which follows a previous lever press with an interval which exceeds some fixed value – the 'DRL interval'. Thus with DRL 15 seconds a response which occurs 14 seconds after the previous response is never rewarded while a response which occurs 15 seconds after the previous response is always rewarded. A CS for shock superimposed on a DRL baseline increases responding, at least with low intensities of shock. This increase occurs despite the fact that responding on a fixed interval (FI) baseline in the same animals shows the usual decrease (Blackman, 1968). Again the competing response hypothesis cannot account for the data (Note 9.1).

It should be noted that these results do not show that every instance of conditioned suppression is due to the conditioning of fear. Some caution is suggested by Bouton & Bolles (1980). They showed that the amount of freezing (a state of rigid stillness which many animals show when frightened) correlated well with the amount of conditioned suppression on three separate baselines: bar press, licking and general motor activity. As Bouton & Bolles say their results 'do not constitute a critical test of the motivational account of conditioned suppression. But they do suggest that a motivational account should recognise the possible role that defensive behaviours can play in the suppression of appetitive behaviour' (op. cit.).

It is interesting that Bouton & Bolles (1980) were concerned with freezing. From the point of view of competing responses this seems a far better candidate than responses such as urination, defecation or piloerection. However, if we are to avoid postulating special internal states it is difficult to account for the ready appearance of freezing. The responses to the UCS of shock which might be thought to be available for classical conditioning consist of flinching, jumping and the like. By contrast, freezing only occurs after a CS (including apparatus cues) has been paired with shock. In one sense then, even if we show that freezing is specifically competing with lever pressing, we still have to postulate the conditioning of a state of fear to account for the occurrence of the freezing.

We can agree to some extent with Millenson & De Villiers (1972) when they conclude that 'Pavlov's (stimulus–response) conception of conditioning has never been empirically demonstrated. In fact the evidence ... is far more favourable to the notion that Pavlov's procedure produces central emotional and motivational states, of which skeletal and autonomic respondents are the least important and least reliable indicants.'

The above statement emphasises the motivational aspects of emotional states. Skeletal and autonomic respondents are described as unreliable and by implication to be ignored. Why then should we talk about emotion at all? Why need we go beyond the idea of motivation, a source of simple variation in the strength of conditioned responses? In one sense the answer is that skeletal and autonomic respondents cannot be ignored – and we have already seen that such respondents, especially species-specific reactions, may give us much more insight into the nature of central states than Millenson & De Villiers allow. However, even if we would prefer to use the term emotion because of these respondents, we could still retain a unitary notion of specific emotions by subsuming the concept of motivation within that of emotion.

9.8.   Motivation versus emotion

Bindra (1969) has proposed the idea of a 'central motivational state' (CMS) which combines the usual idea of emotion with that of motivation. Prior to his analysis there was a tendency to equate emotion with the capacity of external stimuli to elicit behaviour and to equate motivation with the internal state of an organism and hence variations in its readiness to perform certain responses. In addition to this there was a distinction between incentive motivation, that is motivation resulting from an external stimulus (the hunger you feel when you see a cream bun), and drive motivation, that is motivation resulting from an internal condition such as homeostatic imbalance (the hunger you feel when you have not eaten for a day or two).

As can be seen in Figure 9.1, both the condition of the organism (e.g. hunger) and incentive stimuli (e.g. shock) are presumed by Bindra to contribute to the generation of any particular CMS. What have normally been thought of as motivational states are presumed by Bindra to show some contribution from incentive stimuli and what are usually

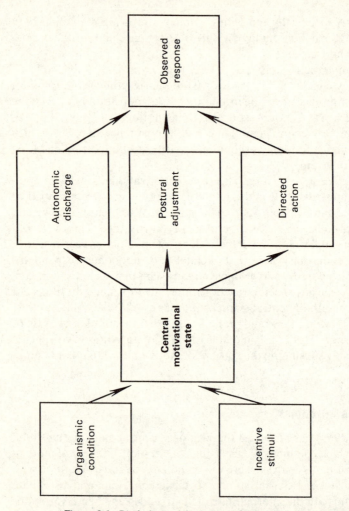

Figure 9.1. Bindra's model of Central Motivation State (CMS). Both the animal's internal condition (e.g. hunger) and external incentive stimuli (e.g. fear provoking stimuli) are assumed to affect CMS in all emotions. Activation of a CMS results in each of: autonomic discharge, postural adjustment and directed action. These then combine and possibly interact to produce the observed response. Reproduced (redrawn) from Bindra (1969) with permission from the New York Academy of Sciences.

thought of as emotions are presumed to have some contribution from the condition of the organism. Thus hunger, for example, would be affected by the sight of food as well as by the length of time since the animal last ate. (In fact there are suggestions that in humans such incentive stimuli can on occasion provide the main reason for eating; Schachter, 1971.) Equally, what are commonly termed emotions would depend on such factors as hormonal balance (and perhaps mood) in addition to the presentation of external releasing stimuli. Bindra suggests that, once the CMS is induced by some combination of organismic condition and/or external stimuli, it generates autonomic discharge, postural adjustments and environmentally organised output. All of these combine as the observed response. So, according to Bindra, what are usually distinguished as emotions and motivations do not differ in their essential control features but rather differ in the relative values of the required initiating conditions. 'This may be a reason why laymen and psychologists alike have come to distinguish between emotion and motivation, but it does not justify any assumption that these are different classes of behaviour or that different explanatory concepts are needed to deal with them.' (Bindra, 1969).

This is a neat simplification of a range of phenomena. However, closer inspection suggests that it is too simple. According to Bindra, outputs such as autonomic discharge and postural adjustment are the direct result of activation of the CMS and it is the CMS itself which undergoes conditioning. During conditioning the CMS will come to be elicited by the CS in advance of the UCS. However, the CMS will still generate the same outputs as before. Thus the observed responses to the CS should be the same as to the UCS. There are two ways in which this prediction appears to fail. First, if we limit our consideration to skeletal responding, we can see that the nature of the response changes as a result of conditioning. For example, (as noted above) the usual response to a shock is jumping, etc. while the response to a CS for shock is freezing. Secondly, if we consider skeletal and autonomic output, we can see that these do not covary in the manner we would expect if they both resulted from the same state. For example, during the course of acquisition of avoidance responding most of the autonomic output, presumed to be generated by the CMS of fear, disappears.

A final problem relates to the assumption common to both Bindra and the position taken by Millenson & De Villiers (1972), namely, that the motivational aspects of central states simply sum algebraically to produce phenomena such as conditioned suppression. It should be noted that, in calculating this algebraical sum, the states themselves are treated as being positive or negative on the basis of their rewarding or punishing aspects in conditioning paradigms. So, for example, fear would in practice subtract from the effects of hunger. It is certainly the case that a signal which predicts shock will increase avoidance responding, a signal which predicts the absence of shock will decrease it and a stimulus which has no predictive value will have no effect (Weisman & Litner, 1972). Likewise, much of the above discussion has dealt with the use of a signal which predicts shock to reduce a baseline response maintained by food. In contrast to these algebraically additive effects, a signal which predicts food does not accelerate a baseline maintained by food. Rather, the animal stops responding and starts to salivate. This suppression is unlikely to be due to, for example, a tendency to approach the site of reinforcement since a signal which predicts rewarding brain stimulation will also suppress appetitive instrumental responding (see discussion in Mackintosh, 1974). By contrast, a signal which predicts food superimposed on extinction of a food rewarded response does increase responding (Estes, 1943). While we may be able to see a number of intuitive reasons for the above observations, they cannot be explained purely in terms of additive motivational effects (Note 9.2).

It might be possible to retrieve Bindra's basic idea of a single central state by suitable additional postulates and arguments. However, it seems to me simpler to assume that emotion and motivation are closely related, but not identical. Thus a particular stimulus or stimulus complex could create either a motivational state, resulting in performance of some conditioned response, or an emotional state, resulting in the release of some reaction such as salivation or freezing, or both. In the examples we have been considering we may suppose that the enabling properties of the central states created by conditioning interact with any motivational properties such states may have. So, if the reactions released are not incompatible with the ongoing behaviour, we see addition or subtraction of motivation (as in conditioned suppression). If they are incompatible, what we see will depend on the interaction of released and motivated behaviour as with the signal which predicts food superimposed on a food baseline.

9.9.   Emotion as a critical aspect of instrumental conditioning

It appears from the above that emotional states can enhance or retard conditioning depending on the compatibility of their releasing properties with the required responding. It may be that the involvement of emotion in conditioning runs deeper than this – and that emotion contributes directly to reinforcement in the early stages of learning. This is demonstrated by two experiments performed by Kamin, Brimer & Black (1963). They first gave rats varying amounts of training with either classical CS–shock pairings or with signalled instrumental avoidance of shock. They then separately tested the CSs used for their capacity to inhibit responding on a food baseline. They found that suppression was a uniformly increasing function of classical CS–shock trials, but that it was initially an increasing and then (by 27 avoidance trials) a decreasing function of avoidance trials. This suggests that fear as measured by conditioned suppression is most important during the acquisition of avoidance responding and is less important as the response becomes habitual. Similarly, Sheffield & Temmer (1950) found that the strength of an avoidance response (as opposed to its probability) increased during the initial stages of acquisition and then decreased somewhat as the response became well learned.

Starr & Mineka (1977) replicated the results of Kamin *et al.* (1963), including an extra group of 'yoked' controls. In the simple avoidance situation a CS is presented and the rat may receive a shock or not depending on whether it makes the avoidance response. The various changes observed in the animal, and in this case the particular change observed in subsequent suppression produced by the CS could be due to either the fact that the animal is controlling the delivery of shock or simply to the fact that the probability of occurrence of the shock has changed. The 'yoked' control is an animal whose behaviour cannot affect events but which receives shocks and stimuli whenever these are received by its paired master animal. The yoked animals in Starr & Mineka's experiment did not show the same diminution of fear with 27 acquisition trials as did the master animals. This shows that the loss of fear with extended training is not just a result of extinction of the Pavlovian CS–UCS relationship (which is, of course, removed as soon as the master rat learns to avoid the UCS).

Is the loss of fear due, then, to the instrumental control which the animal has over the shock? It appears not. Starr & Mineka also found that presentation of a feedback stimulus signalling the master animal's response to the yoked control was sufficient to attenuate fear. This shows that knowledge that the shock will not occur is sufficient to attentuate fear and direct control over events is not critical.

In a later study, Mineka & Gino (1980) showed that the reduction in fear as measured by conditioned suppression was not accompanied by any decrease in response strength as measured by resistance to extinction. They trained animals for either 9 or 27 trials of avoidance acquisition. Those receiving brief training showed response strength no greater than those receiving more extended training, while they showed greater fear.

All of the above data suggest that, during acquisition, but not performance, of an avoidance task, the emotion of fear may make a contribution to motivation. We have already noted that it is only *acquisition* of avoidance which is accompanied by the release of corticosterone and by defecation (Chapter 5). It is also only acquisition of avoidance which is sensitive to sympathectomy. It is possible, therefore, that fear whether viewed as emotion or as motivation is not necessary for the production of well-learned responses.

This type of conclusion appears to be true also for appetitive responses. For example, satiated rats will readily make a response which they have previously learned in order to obtain food, but then do not eat the reward once they have obtained it. The importance of what could be termed habit in the face of changing motivational circumstances is also demonstrated by Adams (cited by Dickinson, 1980, pp.103–6). Rats were given either 100 or 500 trials in which a lever press delivered a sucrose pellet. Free delivery of sucrose pellets was then paired with illness induced by injections of lithium chloride (a control group received lithium chloride injections and sucrose pellets but not in association with each other). The rats' lever pressing was then tested in a session with no sucrose delivery. At the end of the initial lever press training the 500-trial rats were responding at a higher rate than the 100-trial rats, showing that the latter had not reached their training asymptote. Conditioned aversion to the sucrose pellets reduced responding in the 100-trial but not the 500-trial rats showing that the latter were insensitive to the changed value of the sucrose. Testing without reward continued until responding had dropped to a similar low level in all groups. The animals were subsequently retrained to lever press for sucrose pellets. The 100-trial and 500-trial rats now showed equal, essentially total, aversions to the sucrose pellets in this phase of the experiment – demonstrating that the original taste-aversion training had been effective in the 500-trial group. It appears then that, with both aversive and appetitive conditioning, once the response is well learned it may be habitual in the sense of being relatively independent of the original emotion which supported its acquisition. It appears also that, once the response is essentially automatic, the experimental situation may cease to elicit the emotion.

If this suggestion is correct it could provide the solution to one of the problems of the theory of avoidance learning. There are a number of reports (see Mackintosh, 1974, p.333) of extreme persistence of avoidance responding in the total absence of a reinforcer. Mackintosh argues (op. cit. p.332) that such persistence is not universal; however, its occurrence does require some explanation. Given the above data, we can suggest, simply, that acquisition of the response is supported by fear but that after the response becomes habitual it is relatively insensitive to the presence or otherwise of fear, and that the fear does indeed disappear (Note 9.3).

An immediate reaction to this suggestion is likely to be 'but this implies that all responses should extinguish slowly'; and, of course, it is generally observed that appetitive responding extinguishes relatively quickly. However, it is a mistake to think that the extinction of appetitive responding is necessarily simpler than that of aversive. Such a view appears to stem from the behaviourist's desire to speak in terms of relatively concrete events. Presentation of food is seen as an event and hence is easily described as having consequences – failure to present food by contrast is seen by the radical behaviourist as a non-event and hence is presumed to have no consequences. In order to account for fast extinction of appetitive behaviour, we need only note that, as was shown in Chapter 7, omission of an expected reward is not a non-event for the animal – rather it is a highly salient event which can actively suppress responding. This view is not unreasonable, even *a priori*, since unexpected reduction of even a motivationally 'neutral' stimulus can produce a behavioural reaction (Sokolov, 1960). It is unlikely that omission of a reinforcing stimulus would be any less important to the animal. (See Pearce & Hall, 1980 for a formal treatment of the coding of 'non-events'.)

It should be noted that habit (which we have taken to support responding which occurs even when the original reinforcer has been devalued by satiation or aversive conditioning) and motivation (which we have taken to determine variations in the occurrence of well learned response in relation to changes in organismic condition) may be difficult, or impossible, to separate in practice. If emotion provides the basis for conditioning (in the sense of creating certain central cognitive states, as opposed to a simple connectionist view of the type proposed by Pavlov) then it may be that all instrumental responding can be viewed as 'habit' and the concept of 'motivation' can be subsumed into it. Variation in behaviour resulting from changes in the organisms condition could be viewed as complex habits learned by the animal using stimuli associated with its own internal state as cues. To some extent the distinction between 'habit' and 'motivation', once these have been successfully defined, is likely to be a simple matter of choice of terminology. What is critical for the arguments of the present chapter is that the explanation of responses released during the early part of conditioning and of conditioning itself is not the same as the explanation for the regular occurrence of conditioned responding once conditioning is complete. It has also been argued (Davison & Lobb, unpublished paper delivered to the conference of the New Zealand Psychological Society, Dunedin, 1974) that 'emotion is a change in the rate of various responses – verbal, non-verbal and autonomic – which are produced by *changes or signals of changes* in the baseline rate of reinforcement. The magnitude of the changes is controlled by the relative change away from the baseline reinforcement rate, and the changes are transient in that a maintained change defines a new baseline' (my emphasis). Changes or signals of changes in reinforcer rate may indeed be sufficient conditions for the generation of emotion, but it is likely that they are not necessary ones. Further, attempts to relate emotion or motivation to change in reinforcement rate *per se* leave unexplained the lack of effect of devaluation of the reinforcer demonstrated by Adams.

9.10.   Conclusions

The data reviewed in this chapter suggest the following conclusions:
1. that previously 'neutral' stimuli paired with reinforcers (and perhaps other stimuli) can come to elicit central emotional states;
2. that such central states will have motivational properties and will also have enabling properties (Chapter 2);
3. that such enabling properties need not parallel the enabling properties of the original unconditioned stimulus, and may often result in diametrically opposite state-dependent reflexes to them, despite the similar motivational properties of the conditioned and unconditioned states.

In Chapter 7 we discussed arguments which would lead to additional propositions:
4. that such central states have sensory properties; and
5. that the sensory properties of conditioned states need not parallel the sensory properties of the original unconditioned states.

While they are laborious, it is clear that the techniques of behaviour analysis can allow us to make deductions about central states. However, this methodology has not been applied generally. None the less, both the behavioural identification of central emotional states and the evidence that such states can enable a variety of species typical responses depending on the adequate stimuli available suggest that some fairly unitary view of the control of specific emotions could emerge.

It should be noted that the results in this chapter do not entail any simple relation between specific emotions and specific released reactions. The reactions of one individual may not be the same as the reactions of another because of developmental factors. Likewise, both physiological changes (e.g. of the 'prepare for action' type) and skeletal reactions (e.g. aggression) could well be generally released by certain groups of emotions which are otherwise distinct. These possibilities require great care in the design of experiments and restraint in the claiming of undue specificity or undue generality of results obtained for any individual emotion or in any individual species.

10:   Interaction of the components of emotions

We feel, conceive or reason, laugh or weep;

Embrace fond woe, or cast our cares away:

It is the same! – For, be it joy or sorrow,

The path of its departure still is free;

Man's yesterday may ne'er be like his morrow:

Nought may endure but Mutability.

Percy Bysshe Shelley: Mutability

10.1.   Dialectical and non-dialectical interactions in emotion

The previous chapters have, as far as possible, treated the various components of emotion in isolation. One reason for doing this has been simplicity. However, a more important reason has been that, given the likely evolution of emotional systems (Chapters 2, 3), there is no guarantee that the individual 'components of emotion' do not have entirely separate control systems from each other. Such separation would not require us to give up emotion as a concept, since teleonomy alone could provide a conceptual link between different components. However, the normal use of the word emotion implies some direct connection between the different components. This chapter, therefore, considers interactions between those aspects of emotion which have been separated by the previous chapters. Throughout, it should be borne in mind that the usual co-occurrence of such components is no justification for treating them as linked. As a corollary to this it should also be remembered that mechanistic links between components of one emotion do not imply mechanistic links between the same components of some other emotion.

Not only can we expect interactions to occur between components of emotion within an individual organism, we can also expect changes in emotion as the result of feedback from the environment. This is particularly the case when the environment includes another organism of the same species. Let us consider the effects of manipulation of rat mothers before the birth of their pups. It is possible in this situation to obtain effects on the rat pup either directly on the foetus, *in utero*, or indirectly through changes in the mother's behaviour. Such effects can

130

be teased apart by using the technique of cross-fostering, that is allowing a treated mother to rear the pups of a non-treated mother and vice versa. When this has been done, it has been found that manipulation of the mother can produce changed emotionality in her pups when they are fostered and can produce changes in pups fostered on her as a result of her changed behaviour. Of particular interest in this context, the pups of the 'treated' mother also produced changes in the behaviour of their foster mothers. In reviewing this situation Gray (1971*a*) remarks that 'we are forced out of the tidy world of classical science, where there is an "independent" variable which we can confidently manipulate and a "dependent" variable which shows the effects of our manipulations. Instead we enter the confused world of dialectics, in which everything we look at is both cause and effect and the final outcome is due to a dynamic interplay of forces exerted by *all* variables: the mother affects her offspring, the changed offspring in turn affect their mother, the changed mother again alters the behaviour of her offspring, and so on until some kind of equilibrium is reached'. Feedback via the environment, particularly where the environment includes another organism, can obviously add immense complexity to observed patterns of behaviour.

A more day-to-day example of interaction between mother and child is provided by what is termed social referencing – 'the active search by a person for emotional information from another person, and the subsequent use of that emotion to help appraisal in an uncertain situation' (Klinnert, Campos, Sorce, Emde & Svejda, 1983). Given the evidence for innate forms of emotional expression (Chapter 4), it is a small step to suppose that there would be selection pressure for the use of such expressive information by nonverbal animals and preverbal humans. 'For instance, a child does not have to receive a painful shock in order to learn to avoid touching a dangerous object ... a well-timed and emotionally arousing scream or gasp from the parents (suffices)' (op. cit. p.59). More subtle control is demonstrated by studies of the effect on a child's behaviour of the mother's expression. When a mother voluntarily produces approving, neutral or disapproving expressions (chosen from the restricted set of demonstrably innate expressions described by Ekman) 12–18 month old children reacted selectively to the presentation of a novel toy. Similarly, a smiling or fearful expression on the part of the mother will determine in most cases whether an infant will cross to the deep side of a 'visual cliff', an apparatus in which the child is faced with what appears to be a deep drop, but which is in fact perfectly safe (Klinnert *et al.*, 1983).

There are clearly, therefore, a large number of ways in which dialectical interactions can occur between the emotional reactions of two individuals and between components of emotion and environmental contingencies generally.

What components of emotion do we need to consider in terms of internal interactions? The components of emotion we have considered previously in this book are facial and bodily expressions, autonomic and hormonal reactions, directed skeletal responses (of the type for which fixed action patterns are one extreme), and the tendency to learn new responses. As was emphasised in Chapter 2 and Chapter 9, the form of an emotional reaction depends in the first place on the appraisal of stimuli in the environment; and, indeed, in many cases, the generation of the emotion itself will depend on such appraisal. We need, therefore, to consider also the possibility of interaction of specific components of emotional reactions with the cognitive appraisal component of the generation of emotion.

We have, in fact, already discussed the case of one purely internal type of interaction in our discussion of the relationship between physiological and cognitive components of emotion. In Chapters 5 and 6 we noted that peripheral physiological responses could provide the feelings specific to certain emotions, and, in addition, could play a positive feedback role in the control of emotion. Viewed as a simple component of emotional reaction physiological changes would be seen as being released by emotion (or by some aspect of the stimulus environment) and would not necessarily be expected to affect other components of emotional response. What was concluded, however, was that physiological changes do appear to have a feedback effect on other aspects of emotional reaction – most probably by affecting the cognitive appraisal of the situation. One way of approaching this is to note that physiological changes, inasmuch as they generate feelings, can be not only part of the emotional reaction but also can form part of the stimulus context in which emotional reactions are generated. Such a simple dialectical arrangement clearly allows for quite complicated variations in emotional reactions in practice even when the underlying control mechanisms are themselves relatively simple. In the remainder of this chapter we will see that the dialectical possibilities are by no means simple either. Perhaps the most surprising such possibility is raised by recent work on facial expression.

10.2.   The influence of the face on emotions

In Chapter 4 we discussed the definition of facial expressions in terms of their specific muscular components and the definition of expressions in terms of, for example, the Facial Action Coding System. This understanding of the muscular components of particular expressions was put to good use by Ekman, Levenson & Friesen (1983). They used two methods of manipulating subjects. One involved the use of 're-lived' experience in an attempt to generate emotion, the other used what they term 'directed facial action'. The critical feature of directed facial action was that 'the subjects were not asked to produce an emotional expression but instead were told precisely which muscles to contract'. Thus the instructions designed to generate an expression of fear were: a) 'raise your brows and pull them together'; b) 'now raise your upper eyelids'; c) 'now also stretch your lips horizontally, back towards your ears'.

Before and during the manipulations, facial behaviour was recorded on videotape and recordings were made of heart rate, left and right hand temperature, skin resistance and forearm muscle tension. For both types of manipulation, verification procedures were used: with relived experience data were excluded if subjects did not rate the intensity of felt emotion highly, or reported the presence of a second emotion in addition; with directed facial action data were excluded if videotape showed that the facial expression had not been produced as instructed. Verification was found to be important for clear results with these techniques.

Both 'directed facial action' and 'reliving' had as targets surprise, disgust, sadness, anger, fear and happiness – the universally recog-nised emotions. The somewhat suprising result of this experiment was that both types of manipulation produced autonomic changes. More surprising still, differences in heart rate and finger temperature be-tween anger and happiness were similar with both types of manipula-tion. Consistent with the data presented in Table 5.1 (Note 10.1), taking the results of both types of manipulation together, they were able to distinguish on the basis of autonomic measures between anger, fear, sadness and disgust. 'Particularly intriguing is our discovery that producing the emotion-prototypic patterns of facial muscle action resulted in autonomic changes of large magnitude that were more clear cut than those produced by reliving emotions' (op.cit.).

A direct effect of facial expression on peripheral autonomic activity can explain a variety of previous results linking expressions of the face with emotional responses. For example, Lanzetta, Cartwright-Smith & Kleck (1976) tested subjects in a variety of experiments in which they were required to suppress or exaggerate their facial expression while receiving electric shocks. These workers found that the extent of facial response was positively related both to the magnitude of changes in skin conductance and to the reported painfulness of the shock. (The skin conductance effects were generally greater than changes in subjective report.) These results might be due simply to production or suppression of expression in general. However, Orr & Lanzetta (1984) found that a facial expression of fear produced a large change in the skin resistance response conditioned to a tone by shock, whereas other facial expressions, including happiness, had no such effect.

Such effects may not be limited to facial expression. Emotional expression in both animals and humans can include changes in bodily posture – these also could have feedback effects on behaviour like those of facial expression. Gellhorn (1964) reviews evidence relating posture to mood and, among other conclusions, is of the opinion that there is 'a characteristic association of somatic and autonomic processes inasmuch as sympathetic discharge and muscle tone undergo parallel changes under physiological conditions whereas states of increased parasympathetic activity are accompanied by a loss of muscle tone'. The relation goes beyond internal physiological reactions. For example, Riskind & Gotay (1982) placed subjects in a slumped or erect posture for some minutes and then tested them for persistence in a task which was in fact insoluble. They found that the slumped subjects persisted less. An interesting point about this result was that there was no difference in subjective report of emotional state between the slumped and erect groups.

The above data suggest that the production of facial expression (and perhaps bodily expression) of a particular emotion can elicit other peripheral physiological changes normally associated with that emotion. It can also modify the effects of conditioning, but without necessarily changing subjective reports of internal state. In this respect facial expression is like the injection of adrenaline – both can produce peripheral changes which result in changed motor output but do not necessarily result in changes in self-report (see Chapter 5).

It is clear that if internal physiological changes are produced by changes in expression this could account for changes in conditioning (Chapter 6). Whether the physiological changes do mediate changes in conditioning remains to be determined. However, quite how or why changes in facial or bodily expression should affect the autonomic system at all is unclear. It is particularly noteworthy that the autonomic effects produced by expression occur when the expression is generated by instructions based entirely on muscle group. While it is possible that having one's face instructed into a particular position could call to mind a particular emotion, reliving an emotional experience would be likely to be more effective in this respect. It seems, therefore, that we must contend with a direct link between particular facial muscle action patterns and particular changes in autonomic discharge. This opens the possibility of a three step positive feedback loop: facial expression modifying autonomic reactions; autonomic reactions modifying cognitive assessment (Chapter 6); and cognitive assessment modifying facial expression.

10.3. Facial expressiveness as a personality characteristic

All of the above results were obtained by essentially within-subject manipulation. It might be presumed that the the observed link between increasing amounts of facial expression and increasing autonomic discharge would also hold for between-subject comparisons; that is to say, a person who in general showed more facial activity than another would also show more autonomic reactivity. In fact, the exact opposite is the case, with the correlation coefficients between the discriminability of a person's facial expression and his electrodermal response or heart rate response being generally in the region of –0.5 (Buck, 1979, 1980; but see Smith, McHugo & Lanzetta, 1986, for some contradictory data).

Buck (1979) relates the observed negative relation between facial and autonomic reactions across subjects to a more general 'internalizer–externalizer' personality dimension. A negative relationship to electrodermal responses, for example, has been seen with a variety of measures of emotional expression, with a lack of socialisation, with impulsivity, and with extraversion. This last item provides Buck with a possible physiological explanation of the observations. He relates the internalising–externalising dimension to intraversion–extraversion, and this in turn to Gray's (1968, 1970) suggestion that introverts are more sensitive to punishment. From this point of view, the suppression of external emotional responses is achieved through the action of the behavioural inhibition system postulated by Gray – a system which receives input from novel stimuli, stimuli which predict punishment and stimuli which predict omission of reward and which, as output, inhibits ongoing behaviour. 'It is proposed that such systems can account for the data we have considered regarding externalizing–internalizing modes of responses if it is assumed (1) that early in life there are important, stable, individual differences in levels of activity in the excitatory and inhibitory systems; (2) that learning experiences can result in situationally specific changes in these levels of activity; and (3) that activity in the inhibitory system relative to the excitatory system is directly or indirectly associated with increased electrodermal responding and possibly with other kinds of autonomic nervous system arousal' (Buck, 1979).

An alternative possibility is that during development there is a relatively global control of emotional reactions tending to produce some fixed level of peripheral feedback taken as a whole. Initially, then, emotional states could elicit a variety of autonomic, facial and bodily responses all of which would provide sensory feedback. Depending on the conditioning history of the organism, some of these would be enhanced or suppressed. During this process the other components of emotional responses, which were not directly affected by conditioning, could also change so as to maintain some constant level of 'internal stimulation'. This hypothesis would also be consistent with the very wide individual variations observed in the patterns of autonomic responding (Schnore, 1959); in this case, the same argument that has just been applied to individual adjustment of facial versus autonomic response can be applied to individual components of autonomic reactions. It may also be the case that such adjustment occurs in the adult as well as during development.

It should be noted that most of Hohman's paraplegic subjects (Chapter 5) reported increased feelings associated with sentimentality. Both the available objective measures of sentimentality (increased weeping) and the subjective report (feeling 'choked up') suggest a locus of neural control which would be untouched by the lesions. It is simplistic to assume that some simple spinal lesion will remove all feelings of all emotions and, as was argued in Chapter 6, there is no reason why the feelings associated with one emotion should depend on the same peripheral changes as the feelings associated with another. Specifically, if weeping and changes in the region of the throat are important features of sentimentality but not, say, fear then the feelings associated with the two emotions would not necessarily be affected by the same spinal lesion. This suggestion accounts for *intact* sentimental feelings – but why should they increase? One possibility, suggested by Hohman, is that this is a simple correlate of spinal injury unrelated to loss of peripheral function – perhaps a result of the depression which often accompanies such injuries. However, if a balance is maintained between various aspects of autonomic and proprioceptive stimulation so as to maintain a relatively constant level of 'internal stimulation' for the individual then it could be that the loss of much of peripheral emotional responding results in a feedback-driven increase in the remainder. This suggestion would not only account for increased feelings of sentimentality, but would also account for the increases in skeletal responses associated with emotion that are sometimes reported for such patients.

For any given amount of emotion, then, there may be some general overall level of skeletal and peripheral physiological output which can be expected and a decrease in one such component may entail increases in others.

Both the above suggestion and to a lesser extent Buck's hypothesis are speculative – there is insufficient data to make a particularly good argument in either case. However, both show that we can make sense both of within-individual positive relations between expressive reactions and autonomic reactions and of between-individual negative ones. The common feature of the suggestions is that short-term changes in expression and autonomic reaction represent a positive linkage between particular emotional states and the responses released by them, while, in the longer term, other factors may operate to alter the efficacy of the release of particular components of the overall pattern of responses. Whatever the truth of this, it is clear that in considering the dialectics of emotion we must be prepared for different types of interaction with different time courses.

10.4. Autonomic reactions and achievement

Autonomic reactions, on the above view, are not rigid, purely wired-in reactions but rather are plastic and subject to various developmental pressures. While there appears to be an inverse relationship between autonomic expressiveness and gestural expressiveness, there appears to be a direct relationship between autonomic conditionability and more general measures of learning and achievement. Ax, Lloyd, Gorham, Lootens & Robinson (1978) investigated both classical and instrumental conditioning of autonomic responses in school children and related conditionability to the 'Grade Point Average' for each child. Their hypothesis was that 'the aptitude for learning motivation can be measured by the learning rate of autonomic nervous system processes' (op. cit. p.217). They found, on the basis of regression analysis, that of the total variance in Grade Point Average about 20% was accounted for by IQ, about 19% by operant conditionability of the autonomic nervous system and about 3% by classical conditionability of the autonomic nervous system. The autonomic measures, therefore, were at least as powerful as IQ in predicting performance. These results are consistent with findings of reduced autonomic conditionability in learning-disabled children (references cited by Ax *et al.*, 1978,

p.236). Ax & colleagues interpret these findings in terms of an underlying personality dimension which relates to 'intrinsically motivated
behaviour'. Whether they are correct or not, we may note that their
data imply a link between autonomic learning and more scholastic
learning which requires further study. It is clearly possible that, developmentally, the reactivity of the autonomic system could affect
rates of learning.

10.5.   Hormone–behaviour interactions

In Chapters 5 and 6 we restricted discussion to hormones which could,
in some cases at least, be presumed to have a relatively short-term
action which could, therefore, contribute to current emotional state.
In terms of general mechanisms of action, however, there is no reason
to distinguish such hormones from those which have longer-term
effects of a predispositional nature. An example of the importance of
long-term hormonal release, and of the dialectical interactions which
can affect this release, is that of the involvement of testosterone,
oestrogen, progesterone and finally prolactin in the reproductive cycle
of the ring dove where particular hormones allow certain behaviours to
occur and, in turn, the behaviour of one bird can result in the release of
a particular hormone in another (Rosenzweig & Leiman, 1982, Fig.
9-21, p.396, reproduced here as Figure 10.1).

As can be seen from the figure the occurrence of courtship responses
in both sexes of ring dove depends on the presence of the appropriate
hormone (testosterone or oestrogen). It also depends, of course, on
the presence of an appropriate member of the opposite sex. Courtship
itself involves behavioural interaction between the sexes and also
results in a feedforward increase in the levels of the hormone which
initially enabled the behaviour. These increased levels proceed to
enable proceptive behaviour and subsequently copulation. Incubation
of the eggs then produces a rise in prolactin levels in both sexes and the

*Figure 10.1. Interactions between hormones and behaviour as exemplified by
reproduction in the ring dove. Increases in levels of specific hormones enable
specific behaviours. Behavioural circumstances influence the release of hormones. The behaviour of one dove will affect the other. A simplified version
of the interactions involved is shown by the arrows and level of hormone is
indicated by the width of the relevant strip. Reproduced (modified) with
permission from Mark R. Rosenzweig and Arnold L. Leiman (1987) Physiological Psychology, 2nd edition, New York: Random House Inc.*

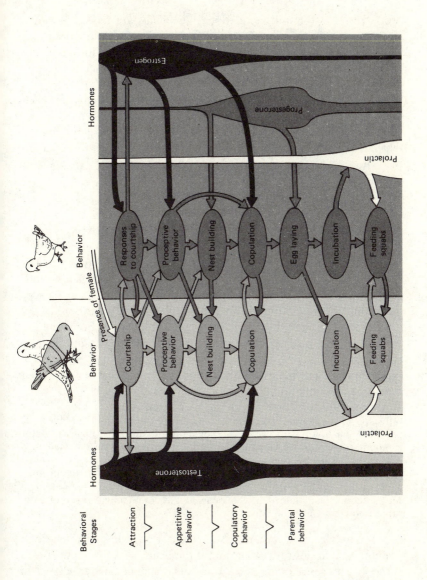

production of crop-milk with which the squabs are fed. 'It is worth stressing the bidirectionality of the behavioural interactions. ... Interventions into the hormonal system affect behaviour and behavioural interventions (such as allowing a female to see a courting male) affect levels of hormones' (op. cit. pp.395–6).

As with the other examples we have discussed in this chapter, each individual component of the control processes involved is fairly simple, but the number of interactions between those components, dialectically, can lead to very complex results in terms of observed behaviour.

10.6.   'Invisible' interactions

The internal interactions we discussed in the initial parts of this chapter are ones which we would not necessarily expect and are certainly ones which we cannot directly observe. In that sense they are 'invisible' to us normally. This makes the detection of such interactions difficult – and, of course, if a particular interaction is sufficiently unexpected, may mean that the possibility of the interaction is never considered.

This problem can also arise with observed behaviour. For example, while females of most species appear to take an active, and interactive, part in courtship their behaviour during copulation appears passive. Appropriate experiments can show, however, that the female is in fact reacting to the male's behaviour during copulation.

Male (rats) normally pause for a while after intromissions, and for a longer time after intromissions that culminate in ejaculations. ... Bermant (1961*a,b*) provided female rats with a lever they could press to produce a male rat. After a mount (regardless of whether it resulted in intromission) the male was removed. The females quickly pressed the lever after the male was removed following a mount (without intromission), paused a bit more after an intromission (without ejaculation), and waited the longest time before summoning a male after an ejaculation. Thus it appears that male and female rats prefer the same frequency of sexual contact.

(Carlson, 1980, p.333)

Not only is this a rather nice demonstration of lust (taken here to connote sexual desire with no moral implications) in rats but it also shows the presence of an interaction between male and female which under normal circumstances is so well coordinated that no interaction is apparent.

10.7.   Some implications for the study of emotion

There are two main conclusions which can be drawn from the brief survey of interactions we have made so far.

The first and most obvious is that observed emotional reactions may be remarkably complex simply as a result of dialectical interactions rather than because of any necessary complexity in underlying control rules. Experiments on emotion need to take this into account if they are to produce clear results. More importantly, theories of emotion need to take account of both short loop (essentially situational) and long loop (essentially developmental) interactions. There is no point in producing a complex account of instantaneous emotional control processes when the processes are in fact simple and the complexity derives from dialectical interactions based on delayed feedback.

The second conclusion is less obvious: that the existence of interactions, particularly internal ones, between the components of emotion provides us with a basis for considering emotions as more than groups of phenomena bundled together for teleonomic convenience. It may be (see Chapter 9) that we will ultimately be able to describe emotions as central states of the organism and that the interactions we have been discussing can all be considered in terms of feedback onto that central state. However, until such centralisation is demonstrated experimentally, the interaction between different components of emotion (where an emotion is defined teleonomically) could provide emotional phenomena with sufficient coherence and integration that even without an obvious central control state we would want to see individual emotions as separate functional entities.

For example, there is no guarantee that a particular *involuntary* emotional expression is generated by the same internal factors as result, subsequently, in a particular piece of emotional behaviour. Yet the very presence of the emotional expression, in terms of its signal value, guarantees a sufficiently close relationship (in terms of probability of co-occurrence in the natural environment of the species in question) that we would want to relate the expression and the behaviour to the same emotion or emotions. If the co-occurrence of expression and internal state and hence state-dependent reflexes were only coincidentally related the emotion label used would merely be a matter of convenience. However, since they are not merely coincidental, and since expressions can themselves produce changes in other components (autonomic and skeletal) of emotion, the emotion label is one with functional significance. Whether this significance will prove ultimately to be that an emotion can be viewed as a specific entity or single state, or whether an emotion should be viewed in terms of a particularly tight set of dialectically linked events, must depend on further experiments.

A final point to note is that interactions may well occur both within components of a particular emotional system and between different emotional systems. Hinde (1970) points out that 'motivational variables normally considered relevant to one group of activities can sometimes affect others also ... . Although such cases have been interpreted in terms of general drive influencing all types of behaviour, it seems doubtful whether such a concept is useful beyond the most superficial level of analysis' (p.212).(General drive as referred to here can be thought of as a simple summation of the intensity of all current sources of motivation – this summation ignores the sign of the motivation discussed in the previous chapter, i.e. fear adds to hunger – which then determines the vigour of whatever behavioural response is produced.)

The complexity of the individual components of emotion, and their co-occurrence, coupled with their likely common teleonomies make it highly likely that dialectical links, both within the organism and through its environment, will be a hallmark of emotional processes. It may be, indeed, that much of the complexity of emotion and the problems of studying it arise from this factor alone (Note 10.2).

11:   Of mice and men

Er schuf alsbald noch andere Thiere. Erster Fehlgriff Gottes: der Mensch fand
die Thiere nicht unterhaltend – er herrschte über sie, er wollte nicht einmal
'Thier' sein.

He immediately made further animals. God's first big mistake: Man didn't find
animals amusing – he lorded it over them, and didn't even want to be 'a beast'.

Friedrich Nietzsche: Der Antichrist

11.1.   From mouse to monkey to man

In the preceding chapters I have discussed emotional processes and
behaviour as if statements about one species would be generally true of
a variety of species. This was justifiable, in part because we can assume
at least some degree of phylogenetic continuity; in part from the fact
that the discussion was aimed at elucidating general principles rather
than specific ones; and, in part from the fact that many of the conclusions arrived at were of the form 'X can occur in some cases but does
not in others'. The problems of making simple generalisations about
emotional processes are considered further in the last chapter.

In Chapter 1, I specifically suggested that general principles would
be most easily seen if we avoided the question of whether any specific
emotion was in some sense identical in different species. However, this
question cannot be avoided indefinitely. Not only does a biological
view of emotion lead one to expect large differences between species in
emotional behaviour (e.g. the species-specific defence reactions discussed in Chapter 9); but also, unfortunately, the question is politically
'loaded'. There are those of a 'creationist' or similar persuasion who
would wish to stress the differences between human beings and other
animals. There are others who have taken it as obvious 'not only that
love and hatred are common to the whole of sensitive creation, but
likewise that their causes ... are of so simple a nature that they may
easily be suppos'd to operate on mere animals' (Hume, 1969, Book 2:
xii). I would prefer to take a middle course and maintain that there are
both strong similarities between the emotions of different species and
also important differences – both of which can only be ascertained by
observation. However, I would maintain that differences between
humans and other species are unlikely to be either greater than, or

different in kind from, the differences which can be observed between separate non-human species.

This chapter addresses the question of the extent to which we can relate findings in animals to humans. In this context both the limits of generalisability and the type of evidence which is accepted as indicating generalisation will be important.

We have already considered evidence both for differences between species and for similarities between humans and other animals. The discussion of motivational and releasing properties of stimuli in Chapter 9 made the case that in motivational terms various appetitive and aversive reinforcers affect behaviour in highly similar ways to each other both within and between species. However, by contrast to motivational properties, releasing properties vary widely from reinforcer to reinforcer. One might even be tempted to define separate emotions in terms of the different patterns of behaviour they can release to identical conditioned stimuli. The only problem with such an approach is the fact that the same emotion can release different patterns of behaviour to different stimuli (viz. state-dependent reflexes in Chapter 2). Further, everything that the ethologists tell us about released behaviour shows that while any two separate species *may* have similar patterns of behaviour released by equivalent adequate stimuli, there is no guarantee that this will be the case. (This should also make us wary of assuming that feelings, viewed as internally released responses, are necessarily similar between species either.)

It is this state of affairs, not to mention its extension to motivational systems, which provides a major justification for Blackman's complaints about the use of cognitive terms to describe animal behaviour (Chapter 9). However, even when observed behaviour differs markedly between species extrapolation between species may well be possible in relation to processes. Unlike the average lion, the average cow does not, when hungry, stalk, kill and eat other animals. However, we can discuss hunger and food in the two species at the level of energy balance with a fair degree of generality.

In the previous chapters we have already noted a number of cases where similar emotional reactions appear to occur in animals and in man. We saw, for example, that the removal of peripheral feedback appears to have analogous effects in dogs (Wynne & Solomon, 1955) and in man (Hohman, 1966); that conditioning of heart rate changes produces similar changes in rat avoidance performance (Di Cara & Weiss, 1966) and in human reports of the painfulness of electric shocks (Sirota, Schwartz & Shapiro, 1974); and that a variety of species including man release corticosteroids in response to the anticipation of noxious events and other forms of stress.

Thus, the cross-specific comparisons which we have already made in previous chapters provide us both with evidence for extensive cross-species generality of some emotional reactions and also with evidence for a more phylogenetically restricted range for other generalisations. We will consider, below, cross-species comparisons in greater detail with a view to delineating both the advantages and pitfalls of such comparison.

Before proceeding, however, it is worth reminding ourselves of the two rather different ways in which the behaviour (or morphology) of two species could come to resemble each other. The most obvious is common inheritance. In this case similarity between the species is attributed to the presence of the appropriate characteristic in a common ancestor. It should be noted, however, that in this case the current function of the characteristic may be different between the two species, and, indeed, different for both of them from the ancestral function. A second way in which behaviour of two species can come to be similar is by convergent evolution – the animals show similar adaptations to a common selection pressure but may have no genetic or specific mechanisms in common. Cases of convergent evolution provide the best clues as to both function and selection pressure. In many cases, common ancestry will combine with convergent selection pressure to maintain common teleonomy of a characteristic in species whose ancestry diverged in the far past. Before proceeding to cases where common teleonomy and common ancestry may go hand in hand it is worth considering the particular possibilities of convergence.

11.2. The lachrymose ape

Humanity has always liked to view itself as above the beasts. In modern times, when biologists have come to accept that humankind is 'descended' from animals, the view of superiority has had to be reinforced by drawing attention to those characteristics which clearly delineate us from our closest relatives, the apes. In *The Naked Ape* (Morris, 1967) and similar works we have studies which focus on specific characteristics of humanity which can be seen as distinct from other related species. Morris's stated intention in his book is to show that humans 'are still humble animals, subject to all the basic laws of animal behaviour'. However, even he sees our nakedness as a unique characteristic setting us apart from a select animal group – the apes. By contrast, consideration of another characteristic which sets us apart from the apes, our tendency to tears when we are emotionally disturbed, can suggest that many of our unique features, in relation to apes, are not unique in the broader context of other animals.

To a Victorian, our capacity to cry might seem simply another example of the finer sensibilities which set us apart from animals in general. However, the modern biologist is left with a major problem – what conceivable selection pressure resulted in this particular adaptation?

A answer to this is suggested by a hypothesis proposed by Hardy (1960) and elaborated on by Morgan (1982): that the specific ape from which humanity is descended spent some time in a littoral or aquatic environment. As detailed below, this hypothesis accounts for a wide range of human characteristics which differ from those of other apes. (Note 11.1) A good starting point in considering this hypothesis is to consider the much vaunted nakedness of man. Theories that man is naked in order to remain cool, to be relieved of parasites or as a secondary sexual characteristic all suffer from considerable problems (Morgan, 1982, pp.27–36). Hardy's proposal is that the loss of hair (or in white people its reduction in thickness) is in response to an aquatic environment since 'hair, under water, naturally loses its original function of keeping the body warm by acting as a poor heat conductor' (Hardy, 1960, reprinted in Morgan, 1982, p.142). As a replacement insulator we have fat, and 'this subcutaneous fat is a characteristic that distinguishes Man from the other primates' (op. cit. p.143).

In the absence of conclusive palaeontological evidence, the number of human oddities explained by any specific evolutionary hypothesis must be seen as its best evidence – the list in this case is extensive and in some respects surprising. Since arguments about precise function can be complicated and are not conclusive a useful way to proceed at this point is simply to ask 'what characteristics which set people apart from apes are shared by people and those species which have adapted to an aquatic environment'? Some answers are given in Table 11.1.

For our purposes the critical item on this list is the presence of tears. Many of the other items, given an aquatic environment, seem reasonable (e.g. the unusual extent to which humans can swim and dive – and do so for pleasure), and have fairly obvious hydrodynamic explanations. Changes in conditionability of vocalisation and changes in brain size can be explained by the increased demands placed by an aquatic environment on communication and possibly motor systems. But crying does not have an immediately obvious explanation.

However, while tears are an isolated anomaly in humans when

Table 11.1. *Specific characteristics shown by humans, apes or species which have adapted wholly or partially from land to an aquatic environment. For aquatic species, Yes implies that the characteristic is shared by several of them (e.g. penguin, hippo, dolphin, otter, etc). Where a characteristic is rare the species showing it is given. The data, in general, can be found in Morgan (1982).*

Characteristic	Apes	Man	Aquatic
Dense body hair	Yes	No	No
Subcutaneous fat	No	Yes	Yes
Streamlined body hair	No	Yes	Yes
Perpendicular stance	No	Yes	Penguin
Webbed digits	No	Sometimes*	Yes
Nose prominent	No**	Yes	Yes
Breasts	No	Yes	Sea cow
Ventral–ventral copulation	Orang-utan	Yes	Yes
Babies born heavy relative to mother	No	Yes	Yes
Underwater childbirth observed	No	Yes	Yes
Midwives	No	Yes	Yes
Sense of smell	Good	Poor	None
Diving reflex (bradycardia)	No	Yes	Yes
Automatic swimming in babies	No?	Yes	Yes
High brain : body ratio	No	Yes	Yes
Conditionable vocalisation	No	Yes	Yes
Speech	No	Yes	Dolphin?
Tears	No	Yes	Yes

* vestigial signs in normal hand and feet; some webbing of feet in about 7% of girls and 9% of boys (Basler cited by Hardy reprinted in Morgan, 1982, p.147); rare examples of webbing of hands (see example in Morgan, 1982, Plate 4)
** one monkey, the proboscis crab macaque, has a protruberant nose – but it is one of the few monkeys which swims and dives regularly.

compared to apes, their presence in other aquatic species suggests that one should look to the water for an explanation. Morgan (1982) discusses this matter extensively with some critical points being that a) seabirds produce the equivalent of tears through their noses as opposed to their eyes; b) sea crocodiles produce tears but river crocodiles do not; c) such tears have a very high concentration of salt. This would suggest that the tear glands which in apes bathe the eyes in mildly antiseptic fluid, could, under the pressure of excessive salt intake, evolve further to excrete unwanted salt – and this would be one of their critical functions in animals such as seabirds.

The tears produced by human emotion have a different biochemical constitution from fluid produced when the eyes water for some other reason. This has been demonstrated by

Dr Frey [who] argues that evolution seldom produces a purposeless function and that tears, like urine, are products of the exocrine system used to carry away wastes – presumably the chemicals produced in the body by stress. It is possible that this mechanism, developed in some marine species primarily for salt excretion, acquired the secondary function of eliminating other waste products secreted during stress and has then been retained in our species (in the absence of salt secretion) to fulfil this function.   (Morgan, 1982, pp. 52–3)

In seals, as in humans, the mother produces tears when, for example, she has been separated from her offspring – and an analogue of crying in response to emotional disturbance can be seen in birds as well.

This view of the function of tears, as a means of returning the body to normal after emotional disturbance, fits with the fact that tears are controlled by the parasympathetic rather than sympathetic nervous system (see Section 5.3 for discussion of the importance of this distinction). It also accounts for the observation of tears of joy as well as tears of sadness – any arousing emotion whatever its affective sign could require a chemical mopping up operation. The pattern of occurrence of tears is also consistent with this theory – tears occur during recovery from emotion rather than at the peak of arousal (see Efran & Spangler, 1979).

Whether one finds this teleonomic explanation of human tears satisfactory will depend in part on whether you accept the aquatic theory on which it is based. I personally find the data of Table 11.1 quite convincing in that I know of no other explanation which will account for it so parsimoniously – but palaeontological evidence would be preferable and at present there is none (although Morgan does suggest where it might be found). It does show, none the less, that a teleonomic perspective can provide quite reasonable explanations (albeit in this case provisional) of phenomena which are otherwise mysterious. In particular, it shows unequivocally that characteristics which may seem peculiarly human when we make comparisons with apes may be, for whatever reason, far from unusual when humans are compared with other animals. Let us now turn to cases where common teleonomy and common heredity may well go together.

11.3.   Separation distress – a general emotion?

In Chapter 8 we discussed the separation reaction which occurs in animals such as rats, cats, dogs and monkeys. The presence of some form of separation distress is widespread. Separation from the mother produces profound changes in human as well as non-human animals. In fact, 'the rationale for the earliest systematic studies of separation in young monkeys can be traced to reports of clinical investigators examining young children who have been separated from their parents, usually because of hospitalisation ... for many children, the loss of the mother even for relatively short periods of time resulted in profound, long-lasting behavioural disorders' (Suomi, Mineka & Harlow, 1983). Children, when separated from their parents, show a clear progression from an initial agitated protest phase, through a depressed phase and then, on the return of the parents, often show 'detachment'. Essentially the same pattern is seen in monkeys of various types with the exception that 'detachment' does not occur, rather a period of enhanced 'reunion' activity is seen.

Thus, while the general form of this reaction is the same across species, specific details can differ. In particular, we would expect the reaction to be less or non-existent as we move to species where parental care plays a lesser or negligible role in the upbringing of the young. Of particular note is the fact that in natural conditions separation from the mother as such may not induce the expected distress reaction where social structure provides a substitute for a missing parent. This factor alone can produce marked differences in the observed behaviour of as closely related animals as bonnet and stump tail macaques (Chapter 8).

The general form of the separation reaction (initial agitation or anxiety followed subsequently by depression) appears highly adaptive. Immediately after separation from the mother the infant is likely to be within earshot; noise and agitation are likely, therefore to effect reunion. If this does not solve the problem, the depressed phase would not only husband the infant's metabolic resources but also decrease the probability of discovery by predators until the mother's return. This suggestion provides us with a possible answer to the problem of the lack of apparent adaptiveness of depression in adult humans. Depression could be viewed as the inappropriate occurrence in the adult of a state which is adaptive in the infant.

Allowing for what can be viewed as minor differences in form, then, the separation reaction appears to be of fair cross-species generality. Other aspects of emotion in humans can be more specific and are frequently identifiable only in apes. The care with which such identity must be assessed is shown by the attempts to identify homologues in other primates of human expressions.

11.4.   Where do the innate human expressions come from?

Given what is known about evolution in general, we can presume that innate human expressions reflect modification of ancestral behavioural patterns. Where such modification is minimal, in both human and some other species, the possession of a common ancestor can result in a similar expression in both species. For example, both humans and apes stamp their feet and bare their teeth when enraged. 'The baring of the teeth is especially interesting. Baboons, which are equipped with particularly long upper canines, pull their lower lips down at the far corners when threatening, so that the canines are exposed to their full extent. We do just the same, although we do not possess long upper canines. Thus the motor pattern has outlived the reduction in size of the organ which was originally displayed' (Figure 11.1; Eibl-Eibesfeldt, 1971).

In the above example both the context in which the expression occurs in the two species and the form of the expression appear fairly well defined. Both of these aspects of expression need to be treated with some care. When we wish to attribute a common phylogenetic origin to expressions in two different species it is not sufficient that the expressions *appear* superficially similar – they must also be generated by essentially the same musculature and be generated in contexts which can be related one to the other.

Consider the status of the human smile. People bare their upper and lower teeth when they are extremely amused. On superficial visual inspection the closest equivalent in the primate repertoire is what is termed the 'grimace', or 'silent bared-teeth face'. 'The structural features of the grimace appear to be relatively uniform in most taxa of non-human primates. The teeth are exposed prominently as the corners of the mouth and lips are retracted; in more extreme forms, the ears may be flattened, the brows raised, and the head drawn back on the shoulder' (Redican, 1982). One of the contexts in which this expression appears is when two members of a group meet each other after a period of separation. It is obviously tempting to equate it with a smile of greeting. However, unlike the smile, the grimace is generally only seen in subordinate, as opposed to dominant, animals.

The other contexts in which the grimace appears suggest that it is not a homologue of the smile – agonistic encounters and copulation. In the former situation the grimace is elicited in an animal when it is subject to attack or threat. In the latter it occurs in the male in association with ejaculation and then it is accompanied by high-frequency vocalisation. Redican (1982) suggests that this vocalisation 'may well keep at a

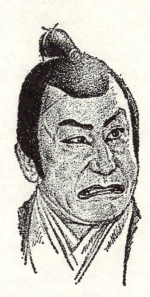

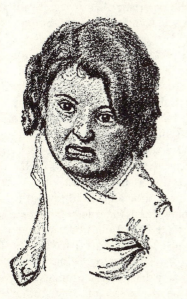

Figure 11.1. Expressions of rage in a mandrill, a young girl, and as modelled by an actor. It seems likely that the human expression evolved initially to bare large canine teeth (possibly as a preparation for biting, and possibly as a display). It has been retained in humans for its communicative value despite the diminution of the canines in our immediate ancestors. The voluntary generation and suppression of such expressions is also likely to be a phylogenetically late adaptation. Reproduced from Eibl-Eibesfeldt (1971).

distance the competing males and juveniles who often harass copulat-
ing pairs at a moment unquestionably crucial to the transmission of
genes to subsequent generations'. Thus, in all three contexts, greeting,
attack and copulation, the grimace may be essentially agonistic. If this
is so, the human equivalent would be the rictus of fear rather than the
smile of pleasure.

As Redican points out, the human expression of fear and the smile,
while superficially similar, employ quite different groups of muscles,
the *risorius* and *platysma* in the case of fear and the *zygomaticus* in the
case of the smile. Since the primate grimace does not employ the
zygomaticus, he concludes that it and the human smile are 'morpholo-
gically quite distinct sets of actions'. As an alternative to the grimace,
Redican offers us the primate 'play face', also called the 'relaxed
open-mouth face'. Like the grimace, the play face is widespread in
primates. 'Components of this display include a mouth that is usually
wide open, with the mouth corners retracted only slightly. The upper
lip may be tensed and curled over the upper incisors, but the extent of
teeth exposure is a highly variable characteristic ... . A significant
feature of the display is its associated vocal component ... that sounds
roughly like human laughter' (op.cit.). As the name play face suggests
it most often occurs during play, and, perhaps most significantly for
comparison with humans, it also occurs in apes when they are tickled.

There is a general consensus that the play face is a homologue of the
human laugh. The suggestion made by Redican and a number of others
is that, in a low intensity form, the play face is also a homologue of the
human smile of amusement. Variants of the play face have been
observed which approximate quite well to the human smile, the social
context in which the expressions occur is similar, and, unlike the
grimace, essentially the same muscle groups are used. Thus, while the
grimace resembles the human smile more at a superficial level, the
evidence at the moment points to the play face as the true homologue.

Primate precursors of each of the accepted basic emotional expressions (anger, fear, surprise, sadness, disgust, happiness) have been
tentatively identified in this way. A possible exception to this is contempt (Ekman & Friesen, 1986) which may thus be either the result of
a mutation in humankind or could be the result of some rather
stereotyped form of cultural learning (but see Suomi, Pers. comm.
cited by Ekman & Friesen, 1986).

Given the specific neural control of expression (Chapter 2) homology of expressions across primates would suggest homology of brain
structures. This could obviously imply that the neural control of enabl-

ing states as well as that of motor patterns would be similar across primates including man.

11.5.   Effects of electrical stimulation of the brain in humans

Many people would find it unlikely that their behaviour could be placed under push-button control. Flynn's data in cats, discussed in Chapter 2 might seem, therefore, to be of little relevance to human emotion.

The study of electrical stimulation in humans is only possible in clinical exploratory operations. This limits the areas of the brain which have been investigated; it limits experimental control over electrode positions and environmental conditions; and it has, of course, meant that the subjects already suffer from abnormalities of the brain and hence may be atypical. None the less it is clear that electrical stimulation in humans can elicit 'movements (which) were not isolated contractions, and only rarely were they integrated into the subject's ongoing behaviour. Rather they were elements of purposive movement which could be somewhat adjusted to imposed environmental contingencies' (Halgren, 1982). These essentially simple chunks of motor output appear to be produced in the same way that stimulation in animals can produce isolated components of particular emotional expressions.

Given the anatomical specificity of Flynn's results with stimulation of the cat hypothalamus it is perhaps unsurprising that directly comparable results have not been reported in man. (The fact that rat killing is not part of the normal human repertoire could also have something to do with this.) The available data on hypothalamic stimulation in man show a wide variety of effects including many non-emotional ones (Iacono & Nashold, 1982). It seems likely that better control of both electrode position and adequate stimuli will be required before we can assess the extent to which human and cat hypothalamic stimulation are equivalent.

The effects found by Delgado with stimulation of the amygdala of monkeys, however, have remarkably close parallels in some human patients. Such stimulation can induce aggression which is directed. The questions of adequate stimuli and social context which were important in monkeys also arise. The patient might tear a stack of paper into shreds but give her scarf into the safekeeping of the experimenter to prevent herself tearing it. Delgado (1969) remarks that 'it is notable that although the patients seemed out of control ... they did not attack the interviewer, indicating that they were aware of their social situation. This finding is reminiscent of the behaviour of stimulated monkeys who directed their aggressiveness according to previous experience and social rank'.

Finally, as we might expect, human beings show individual differences in their neural pathways. These may be more far reaching than those described in the cat by Adamec & Stark-Adamec (1983; Section 2.7) since in many cases the personality of the stimulated subject appears to determine the effects of stimulation to a greater extent than the supposed site of stimulation. The effects of stimulation can also vary depending on the person's mental state at the time of stimulation. This latter effect can even be obtained with simple sensory hallucinations induced by stimulation and is not, therefore, tied to emotional responses (see Halgren, 1982).

This context-specificity of the effects of stimulation leaves open the questions of how far the stimulation directly elicits either an emotion or a type of state which can enable state-dependent reflexes. Delgado's elicitation of aggression might seem a clear example of the elicitation of an emotion; but this can be viewed as the elicitation of the consequences of an emotion such as fear or frustration rather than elicitation of the emotion itself. Equally, stimulation of a wide variety of sites may produce fear or anxiety (see Halgren, 1982), but this could easily be the result of the production of peripheral physiological reactions which are then interpreted in the negative context of the clinic as fear in much the same way as the effects of injection of adrenaline can be so interpreted (see Chapter 5). More generally any unexpected change in physical sensations or mental functioning, even if it is not intrinsically fear generating, could generate fear simply because of its unexpectedness.

None the less, the data we have considered so far are at least consistent with the idea that the organisation of the human brain and the effects of appropriate electrical stimulation of the human brain are essentially similar to those of other primates. It seems reasonable, therefore, to apply the concepts of release and state-dependent reflex fairly generally. It should be emphasised, however, that these concepts are intended to be applied to the *organisation* of the control of emotional behaviour. Their application should not be taken to prejudge the question of whether (Chapter 12) an emotion can be viewed as a releaser. Neither would it imply that individual state-dependent reflexes, or the released responses which accompany a particular emotional state, have control mechanisms which are either unitary or even loosely integrated. Individual released reactions, which we might treat as part of a particular emotion, could well be causally independent of other reactions comprising the same emotion. It should also be emphasised that apparently similar examples of released response in different species should be tested for functional similarity before identity can be assumed. The necessity for this is exemplified by data on emotional defecation.

11.6. If rats are like little furry men, are mice like diminutive rats?

Emotional defecation is an interesting response in that it provides a quantifiable external measure of what is essentially autonomic reactivity. Gray (1987) has made the case that defecation is reliably elicited in animals such as rats in response to fear and, notably, in response to the open field test (Hall, 1934*a*,*b*, 1941). (In the open field test an animal is placed in a large novel arena, usually with bright lighting and loud noise, and its behaviour, particularly ambulation and defecation are noted for a brief period, in rats typically 4 minutes per day on four successive days.) Open field defecation has been used as a measure of 'emotionality' (see below). However, fear is not the only state which could give rise to defecation nor, in fear-provoking situations is fear the only determinant of the amount of defecation elicited by the experimental situation (Russell, 1973; Becker, 1969). One might, therefore, expect considerable interspecific variability in such defecation.

Evidence of emotional defecation has been found in a wide variety of species including rats; dogs (Solomon, Kamin & Wynne, 1953); pigs (Buchenauer, Luft, & Grauvogl, 1982); monkeys (Brady, 1975*b*); chickens (see Candland & Nagy, 1969); and men (Table 11.2).

Table 11.2 *Reports of various symptoms experienced by humans in situations in which they are likely to have been anticipating aversive events (adapted from Stouffer, Lumsdaine, Lumsdaine, Williams, Smith, Janis, Star & Cottrell, 1949; Shaffer, 1947). Note that the pattern of the results suggests that bombardment is the more stressful experience and that defecation occurs with high levels of fear relative to the other measures.*

	Defecation	Sickness	Palpitations
Soldiers under fire	*21%*	*57%*	*84%*
Aircrew in combat	*5%*	*38%*	*89%*

The occurrence of defecation specifically in the open field is less general. Species such as squirrel monkey and cat (Candland & Nagy, 1969) do not defecate in the open field at all. We can account for this lack of response in two ways while retaining the assumption that fear, or some equivalent state, releases defecation.

A first possibility is that the open field produces very different levels of fear in different species. There is evidence that a particularly high level of fear is generally required to elicit defecation. For example, Hunt & Otis (1953) found that, in rats, defecation disappeared during extinction of conditioned suppression well before other measures of the conditioned emotional response. Similarly the data we have on human beings (Table 11.2) also suggest that in humans defecation is one of the least easily elicited peripheral indicators of fear. Species that do not defecate in the open field may not be frightened by it to the same extent as rats and may, therefore, not defecate.

A second possibility is that animals which do not defecate in the open field have an equivalent central state of fear to those which do, but show a generally lesser peripheral response. This possibility is suggested by results with the specially bred 'Maudsley' strains of rat. These strains were selected purely on the basis of their defecation scores in the open field. Maudsley 'reactive' (MR) rats show slightly higher defecation than the original breeding stock while Maudsley non-reactive (MNR) rats do not defecate at all in the open field. These strains of rat differ not only on the defecation score which was used as a basis for their selection, but also in a variety of learning tasks. This suggests that they may actually differ on some underlying factor of fearfulness. Strictly, however, the selection was for 'emotionality' (see Gray, 1987; Broadhurst, 1960; Royce, 1977; Whimbey & Denenberg, 1967; Walsh & Cummins, 1976 and also Section 11.9 below) rather than fearfulness, and the question arises as to whether these are identical (if they are, then one or the other term should be discontinued).

Broadhurst (1957) carried out an experiment to test the Yerkes–Dodson Law in the Maudsley reactive and nonreactive strains of rat. This law states that optimum motivation for performance of a response decreases with increasing task difficulty. Broadhurst tested his rats in an underwater maze task in which level of motivation was manipulated by detaining the animals underwater for different lengths of time before they could start swimming. The task was to swim to the brighter of two arms and the task difficulty was manipulated by adjusting the level of brightness of the dimmer arm to make it more or less like the correct arm. He confirmed the Yerkes–Dodson law in both groups of rats. The important question for our present purpose, however, is whether strain of rat (differing in emotionality and hence, potentially, fearfulness) would affect responding in a similar manner to air deprivation (greater air deprivation producing greater motivation, i.e. greater fear).

The critical results are presented, diagrammatically in Figure 11.2. If the genetic difference between the MR and MNR groups was simply one of the extent to which any fear-inducing condition actually produced fear, then all that should be needed to make an MNR rat like an MR rat is to increase its motivation. In fact, the data show that an increase in emotionality is not entirely equivalent to an increase in fear.

We do not yet have a clear picture of the exact nature of emotionality. However, we may hypothesise that the Yerkes–Dodson law could depend on some single source of motivation (in this case fear) acting on two separate output systems. One such system is that on which good performance depends; the second such system is that which, at high levels of fear, leads to poor performance. If this suggestion is correct then emotionality would represent a component of the first, but not the second such system. Whether or not this is the case Broadhurst's data suggest that emotionality is 'downstream' from, and hence not identical to, the generation of fear.

Mice, however, can not be fitted simply into the above scheme. Although they do defecate in the open field, they show increasing rather than decreasing defecation across test days (Candland & Nagy, 1969; Collins, 1966). Thus, in mice at least, some of the observed open field defecation could be the result of a process such as territorial marking (Note 11.2). The use of defecation for marking is seen in other species such as the Indian musk shrew (Balakrishnan & Alexander, 1976) and the Degus (Kleiman, 1975).

A pedant could argue, even here, that the defecation of the mouse is emotional. Territorial marking is designed to scare away rivals. The mouse could defecate because of fear of the anticipated rival, and the expectation of the appearance of a rival could well increase with time! However, while it is tempting to try and account for mouse defecation in terms of a single factor, it is difficult to do so without *ad hoc* argument. We should bear in mind that, even in rats in the open field, test–retest reliability for defecation represents only about 60% of the variance. This suggests that a variety of factors in addition to fear are likely to be involved in this response.

The above data show that even when we have a relatively unambiguous measure, such as defecation, elicited by similar situations in a

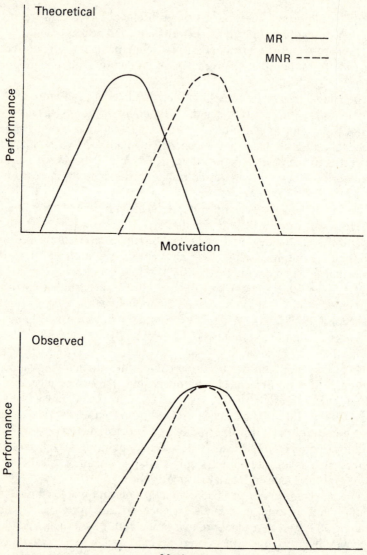

Figure 11.2. Diagrammatic representation of the conclusion to be drawn from Broadhurst's analysis of the effects on performance of increasing levels of motivation in MR and MNR rats. The original theoretical position was that MR and MNR rats differ in terms of fearfulness. The THEORETICAL graph shows one inverted U, Yerkes–Dodson, function for the relation between PERFORMANCE and MOTIVATION (measured in terms of minutes of imposed air deprivation not in terms of internal reactions of the animal) for

range of species, we need to be wary of interspecific variation. However, it should be noted that such problems as we have encountered with interspecific generalisation of emotional defecation are a result of unsatisfactory characterisation of the data within the individual species. In fact, the interspecific generality of some of the observations is possibly the best reason for taking a measure such as defecation as a serious indicator of some internal factor such as emotionality in the rat. It is also of interest that in this case the similarities between rat and human could well prove, once the exact processes and parameters involved have been elucidated, to be greater than those between the phylogenetically closer rat and mouse.

The importance of determining similarities between species in terms of processes, as opposed to in terms of superficial behaviour, is exemplified by data on the partial reinforcement effect in humans.

11.7. Is there frustration in rats and humans?

It may seem surprising that the idea of frustration should require validation in humans. However, this concept was developed and used in Chapter 7 on the basis of specific responses observed mainly in rats. There is no guarantee that the same response patterns will be observed in humans or that particular response similarities will reflect analogous underlying processes.

There are two basic types of test through which a human analogy with the rat data has been drawn. The first, and most comparable, is the observation of responses on manipulanda such as levers and push-buttons. The second, less comparable, is based on performance in paired associate learning tasks.

The demonstration of unconditioned frustration in rats (Chapter 7) depended on the fact that omission of an expected reward in rats can result in more energetic responding, and in the release of aggressive responses. Aggression is also reliably elicited in rats by stimuli such as

(Figure 11.2 continued)
the MR and MNR animals. The curves are identical except that the curve for the MNR rats is shifted to the right because of the lower internal level of fear which is presumed to be engendered by any specific amount of air deprivation. The OBSERVED curve presents diagrammatically the conclusion of the experiment: that rather than differing in terms of fearfulness the MR rats have an equivalent peak of the performance–motivation curve and show better performance at both high and low levels of motivation. Virtually no other studies have varied motivational parameters. If they did it seems likely that 'emotionality' and 'fearfulness' would turn out to be quite distinct, albeit related, constructs.

electric shock. In reviewing the fighting produced by electric shock, Renfrew & Hutchinson (1983) note that 'the generality of the relationship was established in that it was found to occur in other species, including humans, as well as between species and could be produced by other aversive stimuli such as heat, a physical blow and intense noise'. Similarly they note that reward omission induces aggression in various species, again including man, as do schedules which deliver reward only rarely. The latter kind of evidence supports the view that unconditioned frustration in humans is phenomenologically equivalent to that seen in animals such as rats.

For example, Kelly & Hake (1970) tested subjects who were asked to pull a knob in order to obtain money. An unpleasantly loud tone was occasionally presented and the subjects could terminate the tone by either punching a cushion (requiring a force of 20 lb) or pushing a button (requiring a force of 1.5 lb). During acquisition of responding, button pressing rather than cushion punching was the preferred response. When knob pushing no longer resulted in delivery of money (experimental extinction), this resulted in a large increase in cushion punching. Kelly & Hake suggest that this can be viewed specifically as the release of an aggressive response since in a second experiment in which a door handle was substituted for the cushion, but all other details were the same, there was no such increase in responding on the door handle.

Notterman (1959) showed that when rats trained to press a manipulandum for food are placed into experimental extinction there is a transient increase in the amount of force with which they press that manipulandum. This type of result can also be obtained in humans. For example, Ditkoff & Ley (1974) tested undergraduate subjects on a lever pressing task with force-contingent reinforcement. They used two groups, one of which received a money reward for each correct lever press and the second had money deducted for each incorrect lever press. Both of these groups showed an increase in force applied to a second, irrelevant manipulandum during extinction. Equivalent results were obtained by Blixt & Ley (1969) using a similar force-contingent task in children. They employed a variety of different groups. Of most interest is a group which, at the end of acquisition, was rewarded for heavy (forceful) responses and a second group which, at the end of acquisition, was rewarded for light responses but not heavy ones. In extinction both of these groups showed increases in the force of lever pressing which were interpreted by Blixt & Ley as being due to frustration.

In a review of a variety of experiments with manipulanda and children, Ryan & Watson (1968) concluded that 'non-reward leads to increased vigour of performance in certain instrumental tasks'. The experiments included two-lever operant analogues of the Amsel–Roussel double runway frustration effect (see Section 7.4) and free operant versions of the partial reinforcement acquisition effect. (The partial reinforcement acquisition effect is an increase in the vigour of responding during acquisition of partially reinforced animals as compared to continuously reinforced ones.)

The equivalent of a double runway frustration effect, the partial reinforcement acquisition effect and the partial reinforcement extinction effect (see Chapter 7) have all been obtained in tasks where lists of words are learned, rather than physical responses made (Champion, McCann & Ruffels, 1972; Nelson, 1971).

A variety of other effects in the rat literature, usually classified as 'contrast effects', are related theoretically to frustration. These include behavioural contrast and peak shift (Hanson, 1959; Terrace, 1966) and the depression and elation effects (Crespi, 1942; Baltzer & Weiskrantz, 1970). Behavioural contrast and peak shift are complicated changes in the shape of the generalisation curve of a positive stimulus when a negative stimulus of the same stimulus dimension but different value is introduced. Nicholson & Gray (1971, 1972) employed a task in which children had to press a lever in order to obtain tokens in response to the presence of a rocket ship, the angle of which could be varied between the vertical and horizontal. They obtained generalisation curves about this angular dimension which were highly comparable to curves obtained in infrahuman subjects with other stimulus dimensions and types of reinforcer.

All of the foregoing suggests that, where comparable data are available, frustration can be identified in humans in a similar manner to its identification in rats and its consequences may also be similar. However, in one particular area the data, while superficially satisfactory, are far from conclusive.

It should be remembered that, in the specific case of the PREE in rats, frustration only appears to control behaviour when a 24-hour intertrial interval is used (Chapter 7). Humans have not been tested in an equivalent manner (which may or may not require the same interval) and the effects reported so far in humans are, therefore, likely to depend on sequential memory processes rather than frustration (e.g. Halpern & Poon, 1971). Given the clearly different cognitive endowments of rat and man, it is particularly possible that the occurrence of the PREE in humans depends on different types of rule of thumb from those identified in rats – especially since even in rats a number of different such rules appear to be used depending on the experimental conditions.

Thus, a brief overview of the data on emotional consequences of omission of reward appears to provide satisfactory similarities between the observed responses of rats and humans. But, when our theoretical understanding of the control of the partial reinforcement effect in the rat is considered it becomes clear that we have as yet no data available on whether frustration can produce a partial reinforcement effect in humans. The similarities between rat and man may well depend on the fact that persistence is 'optimal' (Chapter 7) rather than on any similarity of the rule of thumb mechanisms used to achieve persistence. Further, where, for example, control by stimulus aftereffects rather than frustration appears to underlie the partial reinforcement effect we have no conclusive proof that rat and man are using the same type of cognitive strategy. The importance of cognitive processes in the generation of emotional reactions, where the reaction itself appears similar from species to species, is brought out in the next section.

11.8.   Cognition and corticosteroids

In the chapters discussing autonomic and hormonal responses, little account was taken of species differences in the type of somatic reaction observed. Yet the physiological advantages on the basis of which such reactions were originally selected (increased muscular energy, blood clotting, etc.) are general. The reactions are also clearly as adaptive for the modern human as for archetypal mammalian ancestors. We would expect, therefore, that there should be only moderate differences between humans and other animals in their nature. The nature of the releasing stimuli for such reactions can be seen, however, as providing them with some human-specific features.

Increases in cortisol (equivalent to corticosterone in the rat) levels in humans have been seen in response to hospitalisation, in response to a wide variety of test situations, and during such activities as driving, flying and combat. It should be emphasised that the changes observed result not from the stimuli involved *per se*, but from the interpretation put on those stimuli. This is just as true for the rat, who releases corticosterone in response to a stimulus when this is a CS for shock, but not to the same stimulus when it has no signal value.

The importance of the cognitive assessment of stimuli is underlined by studies on parents whose children were dying of leukemia (Hofer, Wolff, Friedman & Mason, 1972*a,b*). The parents fell into essentially two groups: those with particularly high levels of 17-hydroxycorticosteroids during the period before the child's death and those with relatively lower levels. It appeared that the difference between the groups arose from anticipatory grief in the former and denial of the forthcoming death in the latter. After the death of the child, the 'high' group showed somewhat reduced levels of corticosteroids and the 'low' group showed increased levels. Taking the groups together, high levels of corticosteroids appeared to be related to extensive mourning. The differences between the groups in cortisol levels, on this hypothesis, related to the different patterns of mourning. The relationship may not have been perfect, however, since at a 2-year follow-up, many of the parents still had high corticosteroid levels but *reported* lessened grief. Of particular note were a couple whose child was misdiagnosed. Their visits to hospital after they knew that their child would survive were not accompanied by the high corticosteroid levels previously seen in them.

Thus, the release of corticosteroids in anxiety-provoking situations is as ubiquitous in human beings as in other animals. On the other hand, highly cognitive factors clearly enter into the individual's assessment of what is 'anxiety-provoking'. Such cognitive factors can then interact with what are apparently more basic, 'biological' variables.

For example, in a study which employed a cognitive task or venipuncture as stressors Frankenhaeuser, Dunne & Lundberg (1976) found that males had an increased release of adrenaline in response to the stressors while females did not (neither sex showed changes in noradrenaline). This suggests that with some situations sex differences can be observed in the release of hormones despite similar changes in both heart rate and the assessment of the unpleasantness of the task. However, in other situations such sex differences may not appear. Johansson, Collins & Collins (1983) found, during *viva voce* defence of a PhD, large increases in adrenaline, noradrenaline and cortisol in both a female and a male subject. They hypothesise that the normal sex difference is due to the different social roles which men and women may be accustomed to taking. How far such differences are qualitative or quantitative is open to question. It seems likely that PhD examination generates considerably more anticipatory stress than the tasks used, for example, by Frankenhaeuser, Dunne & Lundberg (1976). It is clearly an open question as to how far any observed sex differences are socially or biologically determined.

In all of the above cases the release of hormones can be seen to depend on highly complex assessments of the situation (e.g. whether the forthcoming death of a child is 'denied' or not). In that sense the human response may be species specific. However, it is clear that even with the rat data the release of any individual hormone such as corticosterone is neither a simple response to some physical insult nor is it tied necessarily to any one emotional state, rather it appears to result from evaluation of particular stimuli in a particular way. Allowing, then, for differences in the cognitive basis for the assessment of stimuli in the different species involved (i.e. what they will see as anxiety provoking), it seems likely that the emotions elicited and the differences in hormonal reaction to any specific emotion are not greatly different.

11.9.   Emotionality in rat and man

We have considered so far specific observable (internal or external) reactions which, from the discussion of previous chapters, could be thought of as being fairly simple consequences of emotional states. In this section we will consider the case of what has been presumed to be a personality characteristic, emotionality. The data involved can be seen to be particularly relevant to a biological approach to emotion since the animal work has involved genetic selection over a number of generations and the behaviour of interest is, therefore, clearly under genetic control.

It might seem logical to start such an analysis by defining emotionality. Unfortunately, as with many other terms in the study of emotion 'emotionality' has been used in a variety of ways by a variety of researchers – with an enormous resulting literature. Emotionality in the rat has been defined in terms of open field defecation scores – which might be thought to make comparison with humans difficult since they do not generally defecate in response to wide open spaces. However, as was discussed in Section 11.6, it seems likely that this difference results simply from a lower level of fear being generated by the equivalent of the open field in humans rather than a basic difference in the control of emotional defecation in the two species. Emotionality, thus defined in rats, is clearly a personality factor in rats (see Gray, 1971a, 1987) since animals genetically selected to be high or low on defecation in the open field (Maudsley reactive and non-reactive rats) show a variety of other differences in quite complex behaviour. There is also no reason to reject *a priori* the possibility that such a personality factor is present in humans despite the absence of its most convenient peripheral indicator. However, final proof of homology between rat and man must be provided for man in the same way as it was for the rat: by looking for a pattern of differences across a variety of behavioural tasks – particularly, for humans, those tasks on which Maudsley reactive and Maudsley non-reactive rats differ.

There has been virtually no research undertaken from this particular point of view. This is not entirely surprising since the development of the Maudsley strains was originally intended to produce rats which differed in terms of emotional reactivity and identity of the difference between these strains and an equivalent difference between humans in emotional reactivity was largely assumed. With the more specific definition of emotionality provided by study of the Maudsley rats, it becomes not only possible but necessary to ask what relation such a construct could bear to human behaviour.

Eysenck (1967) treats emotionality as being very similar to the factor of neuroticism extracted by the Eysenck Personality Inventory. There is a small amount of data to suggest that neuroticism could be a homologue of emotionality. For example, Orwin (1969) administered the Inventory to a large group of teaching college trainees. He then selected on the basis of their questionnaire scores, a group of neurotic and a group of stable individuals who were then tested in a human analogue of the shuttle box avoidance task. Subjects were informed that there would be tones and that there would be shocks and that they could do something about the shocks, but were not given specific instructions as to how to perform correctly. He found that the neurotic subjects showed faster escape responses and poorer avoidance response than the stable subjects. These differences in performance mirror the differences one can see in the escape and avoidance performance of MR and MNR rats.

It should not be immediately assumed that emotionality can be equated with neuroticism. Neuroticism, as a construct, was defined originally by factor analysis, a procedure which depends on intercorrelation between items. The results of Orwin's experiment (and others in the literature which are less well designed for comparison with rat data) suggest only that if there is a human analog of emotionality it is not entirely unrelated to neuroticism in the correlational sense. Gray (1968, 1970) discusses a variety of arguments in favour of rotating Eysenck's neuroticism and extraversion axes (i.e. expressing test scores in terms of two new, orthogonal, factors each of which would load partially on both of the original ones; see Figure 11.3). He points out that both neuroticism and extraversion load on to scores from a different questionnaire, that designed to measure 'Manifest Anxiety'. Gray argues that, from a theoretical point of view, scores on the Manifest Anxiety Scale might show a better parallel with rat emotionality than either of Eysenck's original factors.

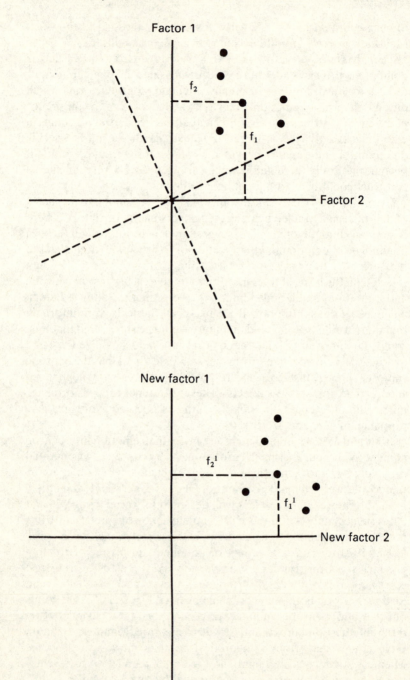

As Taylor (1956) has emphasised Manifest Anxiety is not related in any direct way to clinical anxiety and 'the test might better have been given a more non-committal label'. Taylor discusses a variety of experiments comparing subjects who have high and low scores on Manifest Anxiety. High Anxiety subjects show generally better conditioning of eyelid responses to shock provided that the environment is relatively threatening (see Gray, 1970). This result bears a superficial similarity to the performance of the Maudsley strains in Broadhurst's (1957) experiment mentioned above. However, High Manifest Anxiety subjects have also been reported to show poorer learning of stylus mazes. The Maudsley strains of rat do not differ on conventional maze learning.

It can be seen from the above that suggestions as to the presence of a human analogue of emotionality are totally *ad hoc* at present and the vast majority of experiments on the subject do not address the real questions. What is required is extensive testing of humans on tasks specifically designed to mirror those in which the Maudsley strains differ; or, alternatively, a more conclusive definition of emotionality in humans followed by appropriate tests on Maudsley rats or other non-human species.

11.10. Conclusion

We have considered a comparatively small number of specific examples in each of which we have found a fair degree of similarity between humans and other animals. The small number of these equivalent observations, and the uncertainty associated with the conclusions,

Figure 11.3. Rotation of factor axes: the upper part of the figure shows a set of items located within a two dimensional factor space. Factor scores of f_2 and f_1 are shown for a specific item in relation to the two factors which are represented by the axes (FACTOR 1 AND FACTOR 2). These could be the factors extracted in an initial factor analysis of the data.

Mathematically the location of the axes is arbitrary and the relationships between the different items would be unchanged if we rotated the axes to a new position, as shown by the broken lines.

The lower part of the figure shows the same data points in relation to two new orthogonal factors (NEW FACTOR 1 and NEW FACTOR 2). The new axes bear the same relation to the data points as the broken lines above. Note that the relative position of the individual data points, and hence the underlying nature of the factor space, is unchanged. However, the factor scores of the original item on the new factors (f_1^1 and f_2^1) are dramatically changed.

Factor analysis itself merely ascertains the number of dimensions required to represent a factor space. The placing of the axes is, statistically, a matter of free choice. We may elect to change the position of such axes from time to time on the basis of other data.

stems not so much from an overwhelming supply of counterinstances but from the fact that each species, including man, has been studied in isolation, often for some idiosyncratic purpose. None the less, it is clear that the comparability game needs to be played with some care. The temptation to equate processes across species on the basis of superficial similarities in observations which have not been collected in a comparable manner must be resisted. Equally, rejection of similarity on the basis of apparently divergent observations should not be made too quickly for precisely the same reasons. Determinations of underlying control processes and estimates of teleonomy are necessary precursors to any definite conclusions as to homology.

In my opinion, the evidence is in favour of treating humans as just another species of animal. That is to say, where a variety of different species show some common feature of behavioural control, we may expect it to be present in humans also. Likewise, where non-human species differ extensively we can expect the human behaviour to be idiosyncratic also. Even when there is wide variation among species, similarities between man and animal can still be seen provided the animal is closely related phylogenetically or has been subjected to convergent evolution. Cognitive differences are the most obvious source of unusual emotional reactions in humans. But even here it seems likely that the reactions themselves are ones which could be elicited in other animals by appropriate specific environmental stimuli.

Thus, humans can be viewed as sharing all of the biological properties of other species – including the property that each species has unique features or combinations of features.

12:   Biology and emotion: some conclusions

Another error is an impatience of doubt, and haste to assert without due and mature suspension of doubt...

If a man will begin with certainties, he shall end in doubts; but if he will be content to begin with doubts he shall end in certainties.

Francis Bacon. Advancement of Learning. I.v.8

12.1   What is an emotion?

Each of the previous chapters has provided us with reasons for approaching emotions from a teleonomic perspective and for analysing the control of emotions by biological methods. As I stated at the beginning of this book, I think the data show that biology provides a useful basis for the study of emotion. It enables us to ask the right sort of questions about emotion. I also stated at the outset that the book would not provide a new theory of the emotions. There are two reasons, in this case, why asking the right sort of question does not lead immediately to what could be thought of as the right sort of answer. First, a biological approach should be seen as providing only the foundation for the construction of theories of emotion. (The virtue of biology is that the foundation it provides is a stable one.) There are many aspects of emotion, particularly in humans, which require social/cultural analysis, in addition to biological analysis, for their elucidation. Second, and perhaps more importantly, the biological analyses so far available suggest that insufficient is known about individual emotions, either in terms of their teleonomy or in terms of their mechanism, to justify construction of a large scale 'theory of the emotions'.

Certainly, the arguments so far might make us prefer theories of emotion which have a biological or evolutionary basis (e.g. Plutchik, 1983; Buck, 1985) to ones which have no such basis. However, premature theory construction can lead to two major types of error with material as complex as that provided by emotion. First, to be comprehensible a theory must generalise and this results in statements of the form 'all emotions have the following characteristics ...' or to presentation of theories in such a way that it is implied that all statements are equally true of all emotions. If emotions have arisen, at least initially, through the gradual accretion of unrelated behavioural and physiological reactions, it seems unlikely that simple generalisations about them will ever be true – or that complex generalisations can be made with any degree of certainty at the present time. Second, theories tend to be propounded in an adversarial context. As a result, theorists frequently present us with answers phrased in terms of the resolution of dichotomies. This may make experiments easy to plan but, where a true dichotomy does not exist, it may make the results of an experiment difficult to interpret. I think one of the reasons that the study of emotion has been so confused is that many statements do not generalise completely from one emotion to another, neither do they completely fail to generalise.

In this context it is important to note the explanatory limitations of concepts such as teleonomy. I have treated evolution as an important part of biology. So, in the extreme case, I could be taken to suggest that teleonomic arguments would be the sole means of providing answers to important questions in the psychology of emotion. As I have already stated, I am in fact only suggesting that teleonomic arguments provide a basis for phrasing the right questions and, by themselves, provide no answers at all to the questions of prime interest to the psychologist. This point is particularly important since teleonomic arguments can rarely be conclusive. If they are simply substituted for the type of arguments which have been common in the literature of emotion then we will simply exchange one brand of uncertainty for another – and the extreme difficulty of providing any sort of direct evidence for the historical components of a teleonomic argument is not the only problem in this area.

The usefulness of teleonomy, then, rests not on some privileged correctness which can be attributed to it, but rather on the fact that a provisional answer to a teleonomic question, even if shown subsequently to be partly incorrect, usually provides a good basis for phrasing important questions about emotion which can then be tested experimentally. Even when no specific teleonomic answer is available I think that placing emotion in an evolutionary and biological context will reduce the tendency to make unwarranted assumptions about the behaviour and processes under study. This is particularly important given the tendency of the literature to contain vigorous arguments about dichotomies which often in practice turn out to be extremes of a continuum rather than mutually exclusive possibilities.

A specific case, in relation to emotion, is the internal–external dichotomy with respect to functional control. From an evolutionary standpoint there is no reason why basically similar types of reaction should not be obtained from changes in external stimulation, internal stimulation (e.g. proprioception), either of these, or some combination of both. To take a second case, the different components of emotion could obviously have evolved entirely separately. They could, therefore, have entirely separate control systems which happen to produce, in the natural environment, coincidental responding. The alternative is that some degree of mechanistic integration of the different components could have also evolved. For both internal–external and independent–interacting distinctions it is also important to note that there is no reason to suppose that any two emotions are similar with respect to their control. For example, one emotion might have expressive and feeling components which were elicited by different aspects of the emotional situation and which shared no common control in terms of either stimuli (external or internal) or of internal control mechanisms. A second emotion might well have expressive and feeling components which were elicited by the same aspects of the emotional situation and which, in addition, had strong feedback, or feedforward, effects on each other. Likewise, with peripheral physiological reactions, it is clear that reactions differ between certain emotions – it also appears to be the case that certain emotions share virtually indistinguishable patterns of such reactions. None of these variations should surprise us if each emotional system is presumed to have evolved independently of other emotions and each microscopic aspect of a particular emotion will have its own teleonomic story.

A biological perspective may also make us adjust our views of what should be included within the rubric of emotion. One example of this could be what is usually termed mood. Emotions and moods are often distinguished in terms of the extent to which there is external stimulus control of the state under consideration and also of how acute are any changes in state. However, if we consider hormonal reactions we will see that essentially similar statements can be made about hormonal control in the short and the long term and that, indeed, the same hormone (e.g. corticosterone) may be released either acutely or chronically. Thus, while it may eventually prove useful to distinguish between mood and emotion in some fashion, it is not clear that this is either useful now or inevitable.

So, what common factor can be used to allow us to talk about emotions in any general way? The data discussed in the previous chapters show that there is an innate basis for a variety of components of emotional reactions and that, at least in the phylogenetic past, emotional reactions can be seen as useful. We have identified innate forms of emotional expression, autonomic and hormonal responses, and directed skeletal response. It would be tempting, therefore, to define emotion as any central state of the organism which simultaneously gives rise to all of these components in an innately predetermined form. (This would exclude as emotions any states which did not give rise to any one of the components and any states where the form of the reaction was not largely innate.) The analysis of emotion would then be a simple mopping up operation determining the limited number of different types of central state involved and cataloguing the responses released by each.

Such a simple description of basic innate mechanisms cannot be ruled out because of complexity of observed response or of self-report. Plutchik (1983 and citations), for example, describes a 'psychoevolutionary' theory based on eight basic emotions in four opposing pairs which allows a wide variety of describable emotions as a result of variations in intensity of each basic emotion and the mixture of pairs of basic emotions into higher order dyads.

However, the general course of the evolutionary history of emotional reactions proposed in this book suggests that each aspect of each component of emotional response is most likely to have occurred initially as a result of some specific selection pressure inherent in a particular environmental situation. The complex reactions we see in highly evolved species are, therefore, quite capable of being clusters of entirely independent accretions which normally occur together simply because the separate constraints which shaped them usually occur together in the natural environment.

This is not mere evolutionary speculation. Different aspects of what appears superficially to be a unitary emotional response can be under the control of entirely separate features of the stimulus environment as, for example, the components of the separation reaction discussed in Chapter 8. As Hofer has remarked of this work 'to have inferred that the low heart rates of recently separated infants were a reflection of an emotional state precipitated by disruption of an attachment bond ... would have been wrong and could have obscured other processes from view' (1983, p.204).

This is not to say that any particular current theory of emotion is wrong. I have attempted throughout this book to avoid discussion of such theories. However, the data which could form a solid base on which to build such theories are not generally available. In my opinion it is for this reason premature to ask scientists for even a definition of emotion. 'What is an emotion?' is just as much a red herring now as it was a century ago. How, then, can we study emotion?

12.2. A biological approach to emotion?

The nub of the arguments in this book is that, even in the absence of an accepted definition of emotion, a biological approach can provide us with a means of integrating data on the emotions. We know a large amount about the control of emotional expressions and the physiological changes which accompany emotion, and we can provide convincing if not conclusive arguments as to their teleonomy. The problem of the definition of emotion arises, in this context, only when we wish to decide whether a particular phenomenon is emotional or otherwise. There are clearly communicative gestures which we would not wish to call emotional expressions. There are also expressions which we would want to classify as emotional which can be produced voluntarily outside the normal emotional context. Likewise, while we would want to describe certain physiological reactions (e.g. weeping) as emotional, some (e.g. the let-down reflex), are more difficult to classify and others (e.g. the watering of the eyes in response to onions) are clearly not what we would wish to term emotional.

From a biological point of view, which reactions are termed emotional and which are not is far less important than whether we understand the mechanism and function of the reactions and whether we can relate specific reactions to general principles which are true of other phenomena. It is highly likely in this context that part of the problem of defining emotion is that nature abhors a dichotomy. This is exemplified by the definition of life. It is clear that animals are alive; it is equally clear that crystals of table salt are not alive; the status of a crystallisable virus or components of a chromosome is much more arbitrary – and once we understand the exact properties of a virus, whether we wish to call it alive or not is of no great importance. We can be generally clear about what is alive and what is not, without having an exact definition which allows us to make precise distinctions at the boundaries of the concept.

In an analagous fashion, a biological approach to emotion can separate specific emotions one from the other, in the first instance, as clusters of reactions which appear to have some common global teleonomy or function. (It would not allow us to separate emotions from non-emotions. This would have to be left until individual clusters of reactions had been fully analysed – and, as discussed in the previous paragraph might not be a particularly useful exercise scientifically as opposed to epistemologically.) From this point of view, there may be no mechanistic links (internal to the organism) which connect the different components of a particular emotion. Instead, the word referring to that emotion will derive its content from the fact that the clusters of reactions to which it refers will have in common the environmental or internal physiological regularity which gives rise to their coincidental occurrence. At the least, then, the word for a specific emotion can be seen to refer to a fixed class of antecedents, even if we cannot infer from this that 'an emotion' can be identified as a single state or limited set of states of the organism.

Having said this, it is clear from Chapter 10 that at least some emotional reactions are linked to others by more than the simple co-occurrence of appropriate environmental or internal eliciting stimuli. The different components of at least some emotional reactions interact with each other and can do so in a dialectical manner. The finding that posed facial expressions can produce specific physiological changes is probably the most surprising of such observations – and clearly indicates that great care needs to be taken in any theorising about interactions between emotions at, for example, the cognitive level. But, while it is clear that there would be selection pressure for integration of some initially separate but coincident emotional reactions, it is equally clear that there need not be such pressure for others. It is not likely to be useful, therefore, to define emotion in terms of whether or not such integration is present.

Until such time as the data suggest a more convenient classification, I would personally include within a necessarily elastic working definition of emotion any set of reactions of the organism which generally involved more than one or two of expression, physiological change, innate skeletal response or motivation. (This would tend, for example, to include the let-down reflex and exclude well learned operant responses.) Those who like to think of emotion as an intervening variable might prefer to restrict the definition to those cases where the components interact with each other or where they clearly have a common central enabling state. However, I cannot see that great harm would arise from a broader definition and the complications of proving whether, for example, a single central state is involved have already been seen in Chapter 9. Avoidance of too specific a working definition is likely to be heuristic. As was emphasised in Chapter 1, a strict definition of emotion is unimportant provided there is some other means of categorising reactions which might subsequently be classified as emotional or not. The conclusion is that any particular researcher should feel free to describe a system he is working on as emotional, but if he does so he should be prepared to define its limits in terms of common teleonomies of specific components of the system so far as these can be ascertained.

12.3. Specification of emotions

The same lack of detailed empirical knowledge which makes an exact definition of emotion a chimera at the present also makes the specification of particular emotions difficult unless a working definition is sufficient. Common features of the apparent teleonomy of a particular set of responses may incline one to classify them as arising from a particular emotion, when other considerations may not. For example, aggression has often been treated in physiological psychology texts as an emotion. Even if we restrict ourselves to intraspecific aggression, however, studies of learning would incline us to the view that aggressive responses are enabled by either unconditioned fear or unconditioned frustration and hence should be viewed as a consequence of emotion rather than emotion itself.

In this context, it is clear that the basic expressions of emotion dealt with in Chapter 4 need not each reflect a specific single underlying state of the organism. An expression of anger, for example, could well have evolved to signal that a person is likely to be aggressive quite independent of what we might on closer analysis decide is the 'emotion' underlying the expression. The same is, of course, true of physiological responses where the physical requirements which shape the evolution of the response (e.g. a need for increased muscular energy) are quite likely to be common to situations which differ markedly in their other stimulus characteristics and response requirements – including the possibility that any relevant reinforcers could be either positive or negative.

Whether a specific emotion label should be conclusively attached to phenomena in terms of common response patterns, common central states, common eliciting stimuli or some other characteristic should wait on our better understanding of the data. Meanwhile, we can proceed, as did Darwin, on the basis of comparative data and provisional teleonomic classifications.

12.4. Darwin as the father of the psychology of emotion

In his introduction to the reprinting of Darwin's *Expression of the emotions in animals and man*, Lorenz says

Like all really great scientific discoverers, Darwin possessed an almost uncanny ability to reason on the basis of hypotheses which were not only provisional and vague but subconscious. He deduced correct consequences from facts more suspected than known and verified both the theory and the facts by the obvious truth of the conclusions thus reached. In other words a man like Darwin knows much more than he thinks he knows. ... What is surprising is the extent to which further research, based on Darwin's hypotheses and pursuing them in every conceivable direction, has invariably proved him right on every essential point. ... I believe that even today we do not quite realize how much Charles Darwin knew.   (Lorenz in Darwin, 1965, xi–xiii)

When one great man talks about another, there is room for hyperbole. None the less, it is clear that Lorenz is right in that Darwin managed to make a large number of statements about emotion which are generally acceptable today; and he often made them on what would seem to be minimal evidence.

However, strict evaluation of Darwin's three principles of expression of the emotions (Candland, 1977, pp.45–50) leads to the conclusion that they 'are not singularly impressive', particularly with respect to the apparently Lamarckian notion in much of his writing that what is a learned habit in a parent can be inherited by the offspring. (It has been argued that what Darwin really meant was that, at the population level, a particular class of behavioural reaction must have occurred as a learned reaction before selection pressure could operate on variations in ease of learning within the population and ultimately produce an innate response.) Thus, Darwin does not appear to have been entirely correct either about the facts of emotion or the evolution of emotion. None the less, his answers were much closer to correct than we might expect given the paucity of data at his disposal. I would conclude that this was because he was asking the right questions – those which would give the greatest understanding of emotion for the least experimental effort.

In short, he took a biological approach to emotion – albeit neither involving quite the same biological knowledge nor the same approach as we would advocate nowadays. So what can a biological approach to emotion tell us specifically, as exemplified by the material covered in this book so far?

12.5.   Emotion, drive and state-dependent reflexes

It seems clear that some elements of behavioural control, and probably the control of emotional behaviour in particular, can be described in terms of state-dependent reflexes. That is to say a particular organismic state enables a variety of motor programs and the observed behaviour then depends on the presence of adequate stimuli in the environment to release specific behaviour. Given the command neuron model suggested by Roberts (Section 2.8 and Figure 2.1), it is possible that a particular enabling state, if raised to sufficient intensity, could produce behaviour even in the absence of the normal adequate stimuli. The most likely mechanism for such an effect would be through generalisation to stimuli within the environment from the normal adequate stimuli (cf. the effects of stimulation on sensory field in Chapter 2). The command neuron model also suggests, given the conventional view of emotion, that certain stimuli could reliably elicit certain responses with only a minimal influence from the state of the organism.

What creates an enabling state in the first place? One simple answer would be a change in the organism's internal condition. In terms of Roberts's model this implies a separation between internal stimuli which provide enabling conditions, releasing the command neuron from inhibition, and external stimuli which release reflexes by exciting the command neuron. However, there is no reason to limit the possibilities to this. For example, an adequate releasing stimulus could well be internal, while for a number of emotional, enabling states it is clear that the state itself can be elicited by an external stimulus.

The idea of release developed in Chapter 2 was much broader than early ethological concepts of adequate stimulus and fixed action pattern. The enlargement of the concept of the enabling state to include the possibility that subnormal stimuli can elicit behaviour is close to the early ethological notion of displacement activities – behaviours which occur, usually in response to conflict, apparently outside their normal motivational context. However, the concept of an enabling state implies that both the stimuli involved and the enabling state are qualitatively similar under all conditions; whereas the concept of displacement activity could be taken to imply that both releasing stimuli and the role of motivation can be qualitatively different in displacement activity as compared to normal. In fact, more recently, it has been recognised in the ethological literature that the same factors can regulate the occurrence of displacement activities and the more normal occurrence of the same behaviours (see Hinde, 1970, p.407).

We should be prepared, therefore, for emotions to involve the release of complex patterns of response of the skeletal, hormonal or autonomic systems. This release will result from interactions between different intensities of stimuli with different intensities of certain central enabling states. (Variations of intensity of stimulus, in the sense meant here, can be observed in, for example, generalisation gradients: Section 2.6.) Both the adequate stimuli and the factors controlling enabling state can in principle be the result of either external or internal input. However, some emotional systems could clearly show bias in this respect. We should also be prepared for the functional description of the control of behaviour in terms of intended movement vectors ('goals'), for example, to be relatively simple – while the behaviour itself, which depends on feedback from the individual's specific environment, may be very complex.

12.6. Teleonomy and emotion

Teleonomy can only be loosely related to a concept such as purpose. It is important not to view evolution as working towards a particular goal. However, once evolution has produced a particular result, a teleonomic explanation provides a form of historical account of how and why that result was achieved. For our present purposes, the main implication of teleonomic explanations of emotional behaviour and internal expression is that such reactions have had value in terms of survival in the phylogenetic past – or have at least not been of disadvantage.

There are a number of corollaries of this point when it is put with the notion of state-dependent reflexes. First, complex control patterns are likely to have evolved incrementally. Second, individual components of contemporary behaviour may have initially evolved in one teleonomic context and then have evolved further in some other teleonomic context. Such changes in teleonomic context can be provided either by changes in the environment or by the evolution of new features of the animal's physiological or psychological repertoire. Third, there is no guarantee that any specific component of emotion has any current functional value. (I suspect that 'gooseflesh', for example, is a reaction which would in the past have raised the hair on our shoulders to form a display, but which, given our current lack of dense hair, has no value. The continued presence of the reaction can be attributed to its relative lack of *disadvantages* – it is worth noting that we still retain a vestigial appendix despite the manifest disadvantage of appendicitis.)

We should expect, therefore, a complex mixture of elements of emotional expression in which the control of only some elements is well integrated. Other elements contributing to particular emotional expressions can be controlled independently. Particularly in human beings we must be prepared for systems which are not only imperfect but also idiosyncratic. They will be imperfect in the sense that they are still adapting in the face of current environmental conditions. They will be idiosyncratic since in evolution the shortest distance between two points is not a straight line. Rather, the path taken will be determined by the ease at any particular point of modifying the current version of the system in a satisfactory manner and the arrival of an appropriate random mutation. It is especially in considering the previous advantage to the organism of specific responses that we may gain some understanding of why such responses should afflict us nowadays. Where an ancient behaviour pattern has been selected against, and no longer usually appears in the repertoire of the animal, it is even possible that it will reappear when the more modern response is prevented in some way (Hinde, 1970, p.673).

Having said this, what conclusions can we draw about the control of the different components of emotion?

12.7. Comparison of the components of emotional reaction

Emotional facial and bodily expressions are, at least in some cases, dependent for their form on genetic coding. It is also clear that the display rules in relation to expression (particularly whether the expression is observed or not) are subject to cultural control – as indeed may be their specific form. In most cases the function of such expressions can be taken to be communication of intended action. (Some could obviously retain partially or entirely a physiological role.) Where a specific evolutionary path has been suggested, it seems that expressions may often occur initially to fulfil some specific physiological function. They only subsequently take on a communicative role which may then lead to changes in their form to accentuate their display value.

Physiological changes (autonomic and hormonal) are dependent for their general form on genetic coding. The exact pattern of physiological response in any particular emotion is, nonetheless, subject to modification during development. In many cases it seems likely that such changes evolved to fulfil a specific physiological function, which they currently retain, and which is not accompanied by any specifically psychological consequence (e.g. increase in red blood corpuscles). In a number of other cases it is clear that the physiological changes, and probably the feelings to which they may give rise, have become integrated with the psychological response. They then provide a positive feedback (amplifying) influence on central enabling states (Chapters 5 and 6). There is as yet no clear evidence of modification of the physiological response to enhance some specific psychological function. In general, the function of such changes can be seen to be to place the organism into a state of readiness for some particular brand of action or to return it to a normal state subsequently. Given the delayed emotional reactions in children (which can be taken to imply a primacy of physiological response) it is entirely possible that, with emotional reactions to basic unconditioned stimuli, the innate physiological response to the stimulus determines subsequent reactions to it. How far this could be true of emotions which result from conditioned stimuli remains to be determined.

The directed skeletal responses (motor programs) which accompany emotions have a strong innate component particularly in specific cases and in specific species. Equally, many of the emotional behavioural reactions and particularly the eliciting stimuli in an adult animal are clearly learned. As with facial expression, it seems likely that innate motor programs can be modified by development and learning. This will occur not only with respect to suppression of the behaviour when it is inappropriate, but also with respect to changes in the general form of the response. The teleonomic purpose of innate responses may be presumed to reflect generally appropriate reactions, phylogenetically. Given the complexity of innate skeletal responses it seems clear that, like the other components of emotion, they will have evolved incrementally. This may account for otherwise strange elements of behavioural control. It is almost tautological to suggest that the purpose of learned reactions is to provide an appropriate response to the current situation where this differs from what has been met with phylogenetically. However, the evolution of innate mechanisms which give rise to learning is itself constrained. Innate learning mechanisms are faced by evolutionary pressure to produce appropriate novel responses given the various innate and culturally acquired predispositions of the animal at any particular point in time. For both motor programs and the innate learning mechanisms which can modify them it should be remembered that any regularity of form in normal adults may result from a combination of a general regularity in the environment of the species concerned coupled with some innate predisposition to certain classes of developmental change rather than innate determination of the motor program or learning mechanism itself (see next section).

Cognition and culture are well beyond the intended confines of this book. However, in the context of the previous paragraphs I think it is not too fanciful to see cognition as having evolved in response to the fact that in many cases of trial and error learning, any error is fatal. Thus, means of 'visualising' or 'deducing' an outcome to a fair degree of accuracy are preferable to direct experience of the outcome. Likewise, culture can be seen to provide the products of cognition, or of someone else's trial and error, without the necessity of any hard thought on the one hand or hard experience on the other. For both cognition and culture, therefore, we should not be surprised to find strong links with phylogenetically older mechanisms for solving the same problems.

Having discussed these 'components' of emotion it is worth reiterating that both theoretically and in practice (Chapters 8,10) we can expect some components of some emotions to have fairly integrated control systems while others may not.

12.8. Development, learning and emotion

For all of the components of emotion discussed above we have evidence for both 'innate' and 'learned' determinants of their form. The distinction between innate and learned reactions is one of the most insidious dichotomies in biology. It is becoming clear that even the most regular aspects of higher nervous organisation in mammals result from the interaction of genetic predisposing factors with a regular developmental environment, rather than resulting from purely genetic hardwiring. Contrariwise, in all cases of learning the capacity to learn must itself be innate and other innate factors often play an extensive role.

In what I have said so far I could have been taken to imply that, where emotional reactions are innate, they are fixed and easily identified. It is obvious, however, that the exact form of emotional reaction to any class of stimuli (internal or external) depends on the developmental history of the animal and that with only a few exceptions the actual stimuli which will elicit a particular emotional reaction in the adult animal are learned.

This state of affairs highlights both a strength and a weakness of the biological analysis of emotion. The use of physiological and comparative techniques, and also the experimental control of interventions in the young of relatively simple species, can give us an enormous amount of information about the general principles underlying developmental shaping of adult systems and of the specific mechanisms involved. In particular, we can often show that apparently complex results are determined by dialectical interactions based on fairly simple underlying control mechanisms. In this sense we may be able to obtain a fairly clear idea of what, in terms of observable response, an emotion is.

However, in many cases, particularly with human beings, we are not concerned so much with identifying whether the organism is suffering from a particular emotional reaction or in identifying the exact components of that reaction. What we wish to know is why they are currently showing the reaction and, frequently, we also want to know how to change it. Where an emotional reaction is pathological a biological approach may be of some help; but, under the normal circumstances of day-to-day existence, the 'why' of a particular reaction will address antecedent conditions which are specific to the history of particular individuals or are determined by their specific cultural matrix. A complete analysis of emotion cannot therefore be restricted to biological considerations. It must also include consideration of attitudes, deductions and similar aspects of the person's situation. This will also be true of other animals, although we are usually less concerned about individual differences and pathological reactions in them.

One use of biology, then, is to determine the nature of the basic innate characteristics of emotion and the rules for their modification by developmental processes. It will only be when these relatively simpler aspects of emotion are properly characterised that what needs to be explained by cognitive or social analysis will become clear. Much time can be wasted in analysing the cognitive or social basis of phenomena which depend, in fact, on much simpler, non-cognitive and non-social factors (Hofer, 1983; Schachter, 1980). A premature high level analysis of emotional phenomena may be on a par with the exorcism or beating out of devils in persons whose only evil has been to consume ergot laden food.

12.9.   The way forward

In the absence of a satisfactory definition of emotion, it is worth noting that a large number of questions (for example, whether certain responses share similar control mechanisms) can be answered through biological and particularly physiological analysis without first having to decide what is an emotion and what is not. Also, in my view, quite complex aspects of emotion have been made clear over the last few years by taking a biological approach to the subject. Biology here should be interpreted in the widest sense and is far from being restricted to evolutionary argument.

For example, the understanding of facial expression has been significantly advanced by using scoring systems which reflect specific changes in specific muscle groups and avoid the use of value-laden labels. Equally, confusion must reign where, for example, an 'Autonomic Perception Questionnaire' has no relation to autonomic perception – which can itself be assessed using simple physiological techniques. Likewise, some questions, which would be very difficult to answer by purely behavioural observation, are amenable to physiological attack.

For example, there is the question of the extent to which emotional expressions are under voluntary control. We saw that voluntary and involuntary expressions depend on entirely different neural systems for their initiation. This demonstrates unequivocally that there are both voluntary and involuntary expressions.

So, 'biological' analysis, as it has been exemplified in this book, can be taken to include ethology, physiology, and areas of psychology such as learning theory. Each of these has important data to offer us on the subject of emotion. More importantly, any particular aspect of emotion impinges on each of these areas simultaneously. and, I would contend, should be studied from the point of view of each of these disciplines simultaneously. Ethology can provide details of social and environmental control of behaviour and, particularly in comparative studies, can provide us with clues as to the phylogeny of behaviour; physiology (and its relations, physiological psychology and neuro-psychology) can provide us with indications as to underlying control mechanisms which can give us clues as to the phylogeny of both physiological and behavioural responses; and psychology, and in particular learning theory, can provide us with evidence for internal states and higher levels of control of a type which it can be difficult to infer from either ethological or physiological data. Both the challenge of emotion and its interest as an area of study can be seen to be that it requires integration of data from a wide range of areas which have been traditionally separated. The lack of such integration in the past has probably been a major stumbling block for the understanding of emotion. I would hope that the arguments in this book would help to convince those who study the biology of behaviour that emotion is worthy of analysis, and those who study emotion that a biological approach to the basics of emotion can remove some of the noise in their data. For those who would agree with this in principle, I hope this book will encourage them to go the whole way in practice. It may make the questions apparently being asked in an experiment less earth shattering; but the answers are likely to be more useful and enduring.

The need, in the study of emotion, to cover such a broad subject area has also, probably, contributed to the problem of providing a satisfactory definition of emotion acceptable to all who see themselves as studying it. To say that we have no satisfactory final definition of emotion is not, however, to say that we cannot arrive at an adequate working definition. The definition with which this book started was 'anything anybody usually calls emotion'. I suggested above a definition which was, in essence, 'any state or set of states of the organism which involve the co-occurrence of specific patterns of response of more than one of the skeletal, autonomic and hormonal systems'. Perhaps as good a definition would be 'any aspect of the mind the study of which requires the integration of ethological, physiological and psychological data'! The definition chosen is not particularly important (except that it should be fairly broad) since we have teleonomic considerations to help us. A broad definition of emotion will force us to study an enormous body of data if we wish to understand emotion as a whole. We need some means of dividing this data into manageable lumps. If we define those lumps in terms of general teleonomic considerations they can be made manageable. Note that teleonomic, or functional, argument would define the boundaries of a specific behavioural control system, but would not allow us to decide whether we would wish to call the system emotional. Since, even at the level of the specific emotion, we are dealing with working hypotheses it will not be vital to be certain about the accuracy of our teleonomic conclusions – a change in a particular conclusion would simply move a particular item of emotional expression from one general category to another. It will be important, however, that we should not be dogmatic about our teleonomic assignments. Having said that, it will obviously be least confusing if those who wish to understand emotion in general (which may or may not be possible) study initially those phenomena the teleonomies of which are thought to have been most reliably ascertained. Once a number of putative emotional systems have been thoroughly analysed a grouping of them into one or more classes can be attempted (on whatever criteria seem appropriate in the light of detailed analysis) and at that point a specific definition of emotion, as referring to one of the classes, could be arrived at.

In considering teleonomy it is worth noting the general functions which were tentatively ascribed above to each of communicative expression, physiological change and directed response. It seems likely that a specific expression (as a predictor of a particular class of action) would be accompanied by specific physiological changes (namely those which would prepare for that class of action) and would usually be followed by a limited range of behaviour (which falls into that class of action). However, there is clearly no guarantee that this is the case (as is shown by examples of dissimulation in animals and people), and there is in particular no guarantee of a functional connection of the type which would allow us to conclude that each of the elements of the emotion necessarily resulted from the same central state. However, in those cases where teleonomy is most obvious, I would think that integrative interactions between the components of emotion would be most likely. In such cases 'emotion' as it is ultimately described may have quite similar properties to those we would normally assume. A teleonomic perspective should cause us, however, to look from those cases, once they are discovered, to others which may not be so neatly organised or phylogenetically well developed.

12.10. A specific example

So far I have dealt with observations of specific aspects of specific emotions only to exemplify general points. In this section I will attempt a brief biological perspective on a single emotion, fear, as an example of the type of approach I would advocate. I have chosen fear for a number of reasons. First, it is the archetypal emotion as far as many experimental psychologists are concerned and, within the learning literature at least, seems the easiest to manipulate. Secondly, a multitude of studies in the literature relate to fear and, as a result, more examples in the rest of this book have involved fear than any other emotion. Finally, a proper analysis of any emotion would require a complete book. In the case of fear such a book is already available as an earlier volume in this series (Gray, 1987) – and furthermore, as Gray's book shows, the analysis of fear has progressed to the point where the teleonomic considerations which I would advocate as a *starting point* for experimental research can be compared with the analytical conclusions to be derived from that research.

Gray introduces fear as a state which results from exposure to stimuli which fall into one of a number of discrete classes distinguished by: 'intensity, novelty, "special evolutionary dangers" ..., stimuli arising during social interaction, and conditioned fear stimuli' (Gray, 1987, p.21). The consequences of fear, according to Gray, include the possibility that the animal will fight, flee, freeze, or learn some new response which removes it from danger. But how, you may ask, can such diverse stimuli and responses be related? As Gray notes 'there is ... an ineluctable interdependence between the classification and definition of a set of stimuli and the classification and definition of responses elicited by those stimuli. So ... consideration of the *stimuli* for fear (can begin) only by begging the question of the way in which we recognise the fear which such stimuli evoke' (op. cit. p.27). This is the same problem of definition with respect to fear which was discussed in Chapter 1 with respect to emotions in general. Likewise, although Gray does not state his solution to the problem in so many words, the approach taken in his book is, initially at least, the one I advocated in Chapter 1. His book first surveys the large volume of data which most people would consider relate to fear. He then attempts to generate a coherent set of concepts which can accomodate the majority of the data. Behavioural, pharmacological and neuropsychological data, coupled with extensive analysis and argument allow him to propose that the various stimuli in his list activate particular central systems, each of which in turn generates a variety of responses (see e.g. Gray, 1987, p.263). This reductive approach is, in my opinion, effective mainly because the nature of fear, as determined by Gray, is not too far from our ordinary view of it and, further, Gray does in the end provide a functional account which links the various stimuli and responses together conceptually.

At various points in the book it is clear that Gray's philosophical approach is basically the same as that of the present book in according theoretical value to both evolutionary and other biological arguments. Indeed, he explicitly organises the book into two parts: the first concerned with evolution and development and the second concerned with the organisation of behaviour – specifically by neural mechanisms. However, his teleonomic arguments are provided as support of other arguments rather than, as I would advocate, devices for the primary organisation of the data to be studied. An apparent exception to this is his stimulus class of 'special evolutionary danger'. This is based on the idea that 'where a particular situation is repeatedly responsible for the death of a significantly large proportion of the members of a species over a sufficiently large (on an evolutionary scale) span of time, the individuals of that species may be expected to develop an innate fear of some of the stimuli characteristic of that situation and to avoid them' (Gray, 1987, p.22). But even in this case the principle is derived as a means to account for a variety of species specific responses which are problematic in terms of his other stimulus classes rather than stemming from the use of teleonomy as a major organising tool.

In contrasting the approach taken by Gray with that of this book I shall not be arriving at very different conclusions. Indeed, if my teleonomic conclusions differed markedly from his analytical account then his account should take precedence (since teleonomic argument is intended to provide an initial organisation of the data, a working definition, from which a mechanistic analysis can proceed). My purpose, rather, is to show how teleonomic analysis could have aided the development of the literature on fear and perhaps Gray's own analysis.

Thus, despite my general agreement with Gray's final analysis there are aspects of his approach to the subject matter which, at least in my reading of the book, can be clarified by teleonomic argument. The main points on which I will concentrate are a) the distinction which can be drawn between conditioned and unconditioned responses to stimuli such as shock, and b) the nature of those unconditioned stimuli which can, through conditioning, result in fear. Gray says, for example, 'that one should name "fear" that state which is elicited by stimuli which give *warning* of pain, not the state elicited by the painful stimulus itself' (p.19, his emphasis). This is clear enough and is one way of making the distinction between conditioned and unconditioned reactions to shock which was discussed earlier in this book. But he later defines a stimulus for fear as one conditioned by fear (p.25) and states that 'defensive attack is connected with fear' when he is dealing with 'the unconditioned response to punishment' (p.254). This leaves the reader in some doubt as to what is fear and what is pain in terms of Gray's original distinction.

This problem is a terminological one rather than a fault in Gray's basic analysis of the phenomena. It is generated by shifts between the normal and the technical uses of the word fear. In distinguishing fear and pain, Gray is adopting terms that people will understand to make an important phenomenological distinction. Later, he makes the same distinction in the language of learning theory by stating that 'the states elicited by unconditioned and conditioned aversive ... events are *not* the same' (p.246, his emphasis). Note that we have fear/pain on the one hand and conditioned/unconditioned fear on the other referring to the same objective distinction. I will argue below that this distinction would be less ambiguous if phrased in basic teleonomic terms and also that the more technical conditioned/unconditioned labelling is infelicitous when viewed teleonomically.

Gray also generally prefers to refer to punishment rather than pain (which is rather difficult to define in purely behavioural terms). He defines punishment as 'any stimulus which members of the species concerned will work to terminate, escape from, or avoid' (p.3). On these behavioural criteria a foul odour, excessive heat or cold or humidity, or sickness could all be viewed as punishers even when they are not accompanied by pain. Should stimuli which predict these events be classified as fear stimuli or not? Again, I think that fear stimuli would be better classified teleonomically than in terms of the rather crude aversive/appetitive distinction beloved of learning theorists. The prescription of this book, as a first step in defining the area to be studied, is to inquire about the phylogenetic utility of observed behaviour. In the case of fear as opposed to pain or conditioned fear as opposed to unconditioned fear there is good agreement that we are dealing with a defensive 'motivational system that organises an animal's responding at many different levels (e.g. overt behaviour, autonomic functioning, etc.) so that it is co-ordinated towards the function of protecting the animal from environmental threats, more particularly predation' (Fanselow, 1984). By contrast, I would argue, what we have discussed so far as unconditioned fear or pain must have the function of protecting the animal from the actuality as opposed to the threat of predation.

What should an animal do when faced with the threat, and threat alone, of predation? There seem to be at least three possibilities: avoid detection by remaining still, escape (probably in a stealthy fashion), or prepare some form of defence, possibly with the aid of conspecifics. What should an animal do when faced with the actuality of predation? The two obvious possibilities are: fight or flee – both with the maximum of effort. Note that a) fighting is not likely to be sensible if only the risk as opposed to certainty of predation offers itself, and that b) freezing is downright stupid if a predator has got its teeth in your flesh, while c) escape, if it is possible, is a reasonable response to both the threat and the actuality of predation (although the vigour of the escape might be expected to differ in the two cases and we might wish to refer to particularly vigorous escape as flight).

An immediate corollary of this position is that conditioned/unconditioned fear or fear/pain are not well chosen terms to refer to the difference between the threat and the actuality of predation. While it is true that a conditioned stimulus will usually be a threat, it could clearly, on occasion, be close contact with a phylogenetically novel predator from which the individual animal has had a previous lucky escape. In this case, despite the conditioned and non–painful characteristics of the stimulus, the animal's response should be to the actuality of predation. Likewise, while the unconditioned stimuli to which the animal innately responds will include those of predation (e.g. being bitten) they also in at least some species include stimuli (e.g. distant views of the outline of the predator) which merely threaten. Our analysis so far suggests that these latter stimuli, while provoking an innate reaction essentially unmediated by prior conditioning, should activate similar behavioural and autonomic response programs to equivalent 'conditioned fear' stimuli employed in the laboratory. In Gray's analysis these stimuli fall into the category of special evolutionary danger.

An important complication to note is that, while threat and actual predation (or pain) can be distinguished linguistically and in laboratory experiments, the dividing line between them is difficult to determine in the wild. A predator viewed at a distance represents a threat. The same predator in contact with you is likely to represent predation.

At what distance does the predator shift from one category to the other? The answer will vary even within the same individual at different times. As was emphasised in Chapter 2, a critical determinant of released behaviour is the meaning attached to the situation by the animal. The blending of expressions (Chapter 4) and implied blending of tendencies in the animal also show that the same stimulus can simultaneously evoke more than one type of tendency so the stimulus categories of threat and predation need not be totally exclusive of each other.

These facts should restrain us from using our teleonomic arguments to arrive at conclusions which ought to depend on laboratory data. We have distinguished threat and predation on the basis of the animal's assessment of the situation. Yet the choice between freezing and escape as responses to threat must also depend on an equivalent assessment. How many emotions must we consider?

On the one hand, we could be dealing with a single central state which enables a set of command neurons (Chapter 2) which then result in fight, flight, freezing, etc. depending on the available adequate stimuli. On the other hand, we could be dealing with a large number of independent releasing systems some of which can be coactive. Teleonomic argument raises the question as to which of these states of affairs (or something intermediate) is the case. It should play no part in providing the answer. Its main use is to provide separate categories for classifying behaviours without prejudging the nature of their control systems.

Teleonomic argument, therefore, suggests that in the general area covered by Gray's book we need to distinguish two major functionally separate, if not clearly distinct, types of response (categorised in terms of threat and predation respectively). Whether we should be dealing with two separate 'flavours' of fear (we have already had to dispose of the adjectives conditioned and unconditioned) or whether we should be dealing with two separate emotions (say pain and anxiety) is something that can only be determined by laboratory investigation – Gray's analysis suggests that separate central mechanisms are involved. We can also distinguish, within each of these major classes, minor situational variations that should incline to, e.g. fight versus flight or freeze versus slink away. Whether these should be treated as the results of separate emotions again should depend on laboratory experiment – Gray's analysis in this case suggests that basically similar central states are involved and the variation in response is the result of relatively minor variations in adequate stimuli. We should, as I discussed above, beware of dichotomising states into those to which we wish to apply specific emotion labels and those to which we do not. In all of the distinctions we have considered in this paragraph, both coarse and fine, the animal's interpretation of the stimuli has been critical. Likewise, the extent of overlap between brain systems involved in the different responses does not fall neatly into separable categories. Different brain systems can contribute to different responses or groups of responses to very variable extents.

This point is brought out when Gray makes a case for equating fear and frustration. The unconditioned reactions to pain and to omission of reward are frequently similar, as are the reactions to stimuli which predict these events (see Chapter 7). Teleonomic argument can make sense of this, at least *post hoc*. Loss of food, for example, is in the long term as life threatening as predation. Further, where that loss is occasioned by another animal, fighting will, in many circumstances, be as appropriate a response as it would in the case of predation. In many respects, therefore, we should not be surprised if fear and frustration are similar. However, it should be noted that flight would not usually be an appropriate response to unconditioned frustration and that freezing is not a usual concomitant of conditioned frustration. This seems reasonable given the different natures of the threats to life presented by loss of food and predation. But this very difference makes prominent the question of how far fear and frustration might be expected to be identical, as opposed to superficially similar. We can imagine at least two evolutionary scenarios. In the first case stimuli associated with pain and stimuli assocated with reward omission are subject to very similar selection pressures and hence, through convergent evolution, come to control very similar motor programs or even similar low level command neurones. In neural or functional terms these stimuli could be thought to elicit quite discrete emotions. In the second case a single central state comes to be elicited by one class of stimuli and to enable a variety of responses. Subsequently, the same state comes to be elicited by the second class of stimuli, but the responses are somewhat different in this second case because of variations in the adequate stimuli in the environment. In neural or functional terms only a single emotion might be thought to be involved. Again, laboratory experiments are required to differentiate these potential control mechanisms. It is clear that fear and frustration could even share some functional control mechanisms but not others. How far they involve identical ones I leave you to judge after reading all of Gray's book.

So, in dealing with the general area covered by Gray in *Fear and stress*, we can delineate it from other bodies of data on the criterion of whether the behaviours to be analysed are related to predation either directly or indirectly. Or, we could treat as separate the threat and the actuality of predation. Or, we could expand study to other life threatening situations besides predation. In each case it will be clear what the intended area of study is and how it relates to the broader or narrower choices we could have made. It is only when we use existing terms such as fear that the area of study becomes unclear (and it does so to such an extent that even Gray appears to use the word in different ways at different points of his text). I would argue that teleonomic analysis would generally prevent such confusion during initial periods of analysis of the data. It would also provide value-free (in terms of psychological theory) labels which could be useful even when mechanistic analysis had progressed considerably. As a final note on the teleonomic analysis of fear we should bear in mind that predation does not represent a simple situation, nor one which will be uniform across species. Further, a consistent evolutionary requirement does not necessitate common control mechanisms for the different partial solutions to the problem available to the animal. So, while the assigned area of study will be clear, we should be prepared, none the less, for a less than clear functional separation of distinct components of fear (or separate emotions currently subsumed within the term fear). Even when good theoretical models have been found to account for the experimental data, teleonomic considerations may remain the best basis for referring to specific groups of behavioural reactions or internal processes and may be the best way of relating theoretically derived terms back to conventional concepts such as fear.

12.11.   Envoi

In good detective fiction, while the author may try to lead us astray, there is always a villain with, *post hoc*, a clear motive and *modus operandi*. In real life accident and coincidence are allowed to obscure the data to a much greater extent. The culprit may have mixed motives or there may be a number of culprits with varying degrees of guilt and varying degrees of premeditated involvement. None the less, in pursuing our detective work on the nature of emotion we should ask the same heuristic question as the detective investigating a murder – who benefited? Knowing this will not secure conviction, but it may well indicate how to collect the necessary evidence.

Glossary

Adequate stimulus	A stimulus capable of releasing (q.v.) a fixed action pattern (q.v.), intended movement vector (q.v.) or higher order motor program
Appetitive	Of stimuli or responses – relating them to the appetites (hunger, thirst, lust, etc.), and implying positive reinforcement (q.v.). To be distinguished from aversive (q.v.)
Aversive	Of stimuli or responses – relating them to withdrawal and the central states which can mediate negative reinforcement (q.v.). To be distinguished from appetitive (q.v.)
Autonomic	Pertaining to the autonomic nervous system which controls the functioning of many bodily organs and glands – see Section 5.3
Classical conditioning	The procedure of following a signal with a reinforcer (q.v.) or, depending on context, a specific form of learning related to that procedure – distinct from instrumental conditioning (q.v.)
Central motivational state	A central state of the organism proposed by Bindra which receives input both from incentive stimuli and from organismic state and hence shares the properties both of what is often termed emotion and of what is often termed motivation (see Chapter 9)
Cognition	Those processes which underlie the manipulation by the animal of sensory and memory information so as to produce novel behavioural sequences which are not the result of simple associative information processing
Conditioned	Of stimuli, those stimuli explicitly or implicitly used by an experimenter, or occurring in the usual environment of an animal, which provide information about the occurrence of other events (which are often reinforcers but need not be). Of responses, those which occur *as a result of conditioning* and are under the control of conditioned stimuli
Conditioned suppression	The procedure of pairing a stimulus unconditionally with shock and assessing the result on a positively reinforced (q.v.) baseline. Or, the suppression of positively reinforced responding which results from this procedure. Also known as the CER or conditioned emotional response
Cross tolerance	Used of emotional states in the present book but used in the drug literature for cases where exposure to a particular drug leads to a reduced response to that drug (tolerance) and where tolerance to one drug can be shown to have de-

veloped to a second drug to which the animal was not previously exposed. With drugs, a common receptor or common response system underlies cross tolerance and it may be presumed that this is true also for cross tolerance to emotional stimuli

Dialectical
Mutually interacting, in the sense that changes in a particular locus within a system can be seen as both cause and effect as a result of feedback (within the system of interest or via its environment)

Emotion
Currently undefinable in any strict sense – Section 12.2 – but may be taken to include any item which has been referred to by the word in colloquial or more technical usage

Emotionality
Used specifically within the present book to refer to that personality characteristic which is reflected in genetically controlled individual differences in the open field defecation scores of rats and to the same underlying central physiological properties in other species

Enabling
Usually used in relation to computers – the operation of permitting some action to occur without forcing it to do so (as opposed to disabling the operation). Used in the present book in relation to state-dependent reflexes (q.v.) and contrasted with release (see Chapter 2)

Fixed action pattern
A complex sequence of responses which occurs in the same or nearly similar form on successive occasions and in separate individuals of a species and which is largely innately determined

Functional explanations
Explanations in terms of function as opposed to both teleonomy and immediate cause. Examples of functional explanations would include explanation of the shark's shape in terms of hydrodynamics and explanations of the form of the eye in terms of the physics of sight. Where a functional explanation is also based on a demonstration of the evolution of a feature it is a teleonomic explanation (q.v.)

Incentive stimulus
A stimulus which induces a motivational (q.v.) state or increases the strength of existing motivation. An example from most people's experience is the hunger which one feels on sight of a cream bun – the bun is an incentive stimulus

Instrumental conditioning
The procedure of following a response with a reinforcer (q.v.) or the specific form of learning related to that procedure to be distinguished from classical conditioning (q.v.)

Intended movement vector
A motor command expressed in terms of proprioceptive coordinates. Effectively this specifies the endpoint or goal of a motor sequence. The motor system and any feedback from the environment can combine to produce the final movements observed (see Chapter 2)

Motivation
An inferred property of the nervous system which is responsible for variation in the intensity with which unconditioned responses are produced and the speed with which new responses are learned in relation to the presentation of specific classes of reinforcer – viz. the reinforcer food and

	the associated motivation of hunger
Negative reinforcement	see Reinforcer
Optimal foraging	The notional performance of the theoretical ideal forager. Given a complete specification of the limits and constraints on a system optimal foraging can be determined. As used in this book optimal foraging and the variety of models which can be used to estimate optimality are guides to what might be expected of an animal under fixed conditions or of what variations in environmental conditions could be made without affecting the Darwinian fitness of specific behaviour – see also Rule of Thumb
Positive reinforcement	see Reinforcer
Punishment	The procedure of making a negative reinforcer (q.v.) contingent on a response. Or, the reinforcer itself
Radical behaviourism	The dogma that only environmental stimuli and observable behavioural responses and the mathematical relations between these can be used in analysis of behaviour. Contrasted, in this book, with analyses such as cognitive behaviourism which allow one to infer central processes from behavioural observations – not entirely a straw man as at least one member of my department is a radical behaviourist
Reinforcer	A stimulus such as food or shock which if paired with a response will change the probability of occurrence of the response. A positive reinforcer produces an increase in responding and a negative reinforcer a decrease
Release	The production of a response or response sequence in an essentially unconditional manner. Normally used of the production of responses such as fixed action patterns (q.v.) by exteroceptive stimuli. Used in the present book to include cases where releasing stimuli may be interoceptive stimuli or internal states and where the responses can be intended movement vectors (q.v.)
Reward	The procedure of making a positive reinforcer (q.v.) contingent on a response. Or, the reinforcer itself
Rule of thumb	In the context of Optimal Foraging (q.v.) which can be seen as specifying what the animal ought to do – and which involves very complex mathematics – a rule of thumb specifies a simple rule which an animal may or does use to achieve optimal performance, usually within a limited environmental domain, without the need to solve optimality equations
Sign stimulus	The, usually specific, stimulus which will release a fixed action pattern (q.v.)
State-dependent reflex	A response, intended movement vector (q.v.) or complex motor program which is enabled (q.v.) by an internal state of the organism and which is only then released (q.v.) if an adequate stimulus (q.v.) is available
Teleology	Explanations of the present state of a system which depend on some future state of the system – see Chapter 3. Contrasted in the present book with teleonomy (q.v.)

Teleonomy   Evolutionary purpose – where there is no assumption of any
                      purposive agent. In many cases synonymous with function,
                      but with the added restriction that the evolutionary history
                      of the characteristic referred to is known. For behaviour the
                      best evidence of some common teleonomy between control
                      systems in different species is demonstration of convergent
                      evolution (see Chapter 3). Not to be confused with teleolo-
                      gy (q.v.)

Unconditioned   Of stimuli or responses, those contributing to the normal
                      innate repertoire of the animal (with the implication that
                      such stimuli and responses may be employed in conditioning
                      procedures)

Notes

Chapter 2

1. The term 'state-dependent reflex' was used by the late G.V. Goddard while describing Flynn's work to me. I have not been able to find its use in Flynn's own writings.

Chapter 3

1. In this context it is my suspicion that the aggression released by fear and the aggression released by frustration may involve an identical control system for the generation of aggressive behaviour – but that this system is released by these two emotions with differing teleonomies. That is to say that separate evolutionary pressures attached aggression to fear and to frustration (assuming these to be unitary states – more complex teleonomy is obviously possible). If fear is seen as a response to threat then the resultant 'aggressive' behaviour can be viewed, functionally, as defense against a direct attack. By contrast, frustration, especially if defined as the response to omission of an expected positive reinforcer (e.g. loss of food), does not, on the face of it, require aggression to be linked to it. It is only when we realise that an extremely common source of removal of such positive reinforcers will be the action of another organism, a conspecific, and that a 'reflexive' attack could well recover the reward that the release of aggression becomes reasonable. If the teleonomies of the release of aggression are different for these two emotions, even when the basic enabled motor programs are the same, we might expect there to be subtle differences in either the nature of that release or in the nature of the release of associated, e.g. autonomic, systems.

Chapter 4

1. The balance between conflicting tendencies (in this case the advantage to the individual of truthful communication versus the advantage to the individual of deceit) may be complex and it has been argued that what will be seen depends less on what appears advantageous in the short term than what represents and evolutionarily stable strategy (see Dawkins, 1978, p.74 et seq.).

2. Similar figures are available for cats (Leyhausen, 1956, reproduced as Fig. 16.10 in Hinde, 1966) and dogs (Lorenz, 1952, reproduced as Fig. 15 in Eibl-Eibesfeldt, 1971). All these figures involve a fight/flight blend. It might be argued, therefore, that we have here a mixture of released response tendencies to one emotion (fear) rather than a mixture of emotions. Fear would then be seen as enabling a variety of motor programs (including fight and flight) and then specific stimuli in the environment would elicit, separately, the fight and flight tendencies. It may be a matter of terminology whether one wishes to refer to fight and flight, under these circumstances, as resulting from a single emotion or reflecting separate emotions (of 'bravery' and 'cowardice' perhaps).

196

Chapter 5

1. It is possible that the release of corticosterone in the open field (a conventional test of emotionality, see Chapter 11) is not a result of fear. For example, no decrease in corticosterone over trials was seen by Ader (1969) in a study which found the usual decreases in defecation with trials. This would tend to suggest that different factors were controlling the release of corticosterone and fecal boli. However, Levine, Haltmeyer, Karas & Denenberg (1967) found a decline in release of corticosterone in response to repeated testing in the open field, suggesting a parallel with the decline normally seen in defecation. Unfortunately, it is not clear from their results that defecation itself was declining (they report only percentage of animals defecating, not amount of defecation).

The discrepancy in the observations of corticosterone in the above studies can be attributed to the methods of sampling corticosterone. Levine *et al.* observed a decline in corticosterone only when blood samples were taken immediately after testing. No such decline was seen if the samples were taken 15 minutes after (when levels were maximal). Ader's samples were also obtained 15 minutes after testing and hence could have missed a period during which differential results across days would have been seen.

It should always be remembered that the release of corticosterone in these experiments is consequent on release of ACTH from the pituitary. This accounts for the long delay in obtaining maximal release after the test. One explanation, therefore, of the above observations is that the release of ACTH is decreasing with days of testing but that it is sufficient on all days to ultimately produce maximal, asymptotic, release of corticosterone. The period immediately after testing would sample only the initial stages of corticosterone release and hence would be more sensitive to the amount of ACTH. This explanation seems preferable to the idea that in the open field corticosterone release is determined by some process other than fear. However, since we have concluded that corticosterone release is not specific to fear, further careful experiments measuring corticosterone, amount of defecation, and ideally ACTH at a number of time intervals will be required to settle the matter.

2. One example of the sharing of at least some components of emotional feeling, or physiological reaction, could be the observation of cross-tolerance between fear and frustration (Brown & Wagner, 1964). In these experiments, using resistance to extinction or punishment as a measure, it is found that prior experience of frustration increases resistance to fear and vice versa. Since the cross-tolerance is not complete we have no reason to suppose that the animals view the two states as being identical. Fear and frustration may thus be quite distinct both neurally and at the level of psychological process while having in common some of the feelings (from e.g. release of corticosterone, Section 5.6) and state-dependent reflexes (e.g. aggression) which they release (see also Chapter 9 and Note 7.6).

Chapter 6

1. Removal of the pituitary (like peripheral sympathectomy) retards the acquisition and facilitates the extinction of avoidance responses. Injection of ACTH reverses these effects (see Levine, 1971; Leshner, 1977).

Adrenal demedullation has less obvious effects. It does not change acquisition of one way avoidance, startle reactions, or defecation (Moyer & Bunnell, 1959, 1960*a,b*) although it may have a small effect on shock threshold (Pare, 1969). Effects on two-way avoidance performance and retention have been reported (Caldwell, 1962; Levine &

Soliday, 1962)

Removal of the entire adrenal, like demedullation, has no effect on shock thresholds (Pare, 1969), neither does it affect the acquisition or extinction of escape responses (Moyer, 1958a; Borda-Bossana, Elrick, Bernstein & Atkinson, 1961). Both increases decreases in defecation have been reported (Paul & Havlena, 1962; Moyer, 1958b). Adrenalectomy has been reported to increase responses to fear as assessed in some active and passive avoidance situations and it retards extinction of avoidance (Levine, 1971; Leshner, 1977). However, its effects on two-way avoidance (Beatty *et al.*, 1970) can be like those of anti-anxiety drugs (Gray, 1977) and in a number of cases adrenalectomy does not appear to affect one-way, two-way or passive avoidance (see Table 1, McNaughton & Mason, 1980; De Wied, van Delft, Gispen, Weijnen & van Wimersma Greidanus, 1972). Some variations in the results obtained could be due to apparatus (see Roberts & Fibiger, 1977) or to only partial removal of the gland. An interaction with at least some components of the response to fear could also underlie effects on appetitive learning. For example, handling of animals generally improves their capacity for discrimination learning and adrenalectomy reduces this handling effect (Borda-Bossana *et al.*, 1961). Adrenalectomy has also been reported to produce somewhat complicated changes in the course of maze learning (Paul & Havlena, 1962).

2. This is certainly true for the combination of adrenalectomy with loss of *central* noradrenaline. A number of studies have found that while adrenalectomy or lesions of the dorsal ascending noradrenergic bundle have little or no effect on behaviour by themselves, their combination did have significant effects. This has been found with one-way active avoidance, two-way avoidance, passive avoidance, and open field rearing (see McNaughton & Mason, 1980).

3. Administration of ACTH (i.e. increases in both ACTH and corticosterone) does not affect acquisition of appetitive or active avoidance responses nor does it affect the baseline response used in a passive avoidance task. It improves acquisition of passive avoidance and retards extinction of rewarded behaviour, of passive avoidance and of active avoidance. It produces a state-dependent reduction in the partial reinforcement extinction effect (see Chapter 7). Administration of ACTH only on the first day of acquisition of an appetitive response is sufficient to immunise the animal against the retardation produced by ACTH given in extinction although it does not by itself affect the rate of extinction to a great extent (Levine & Jones, 1965; Miller & Ogawa, 1962; Garrud, Gray & De Wied, 1974; Gray, 1971b; Gray, Mayes & Wilson, 1971; and review by Leshner, 1977).

ACTH is a fairly large molecule consisting of a chain of amino acids. It is possible to synthesise portions of it which mimic its actions to different extents. These portions are usually referred to by the amino acids of the full ACTH molecule from which they are made up, thus ACTH 4–10 is a molecule consisting of the 4th–10th amino acids of the full molecule. Some of the synthetic molecules, e.g. ACTH 1–24, have the same adrenocortical activity as the full molecule while others, e.g. ACTH 1–10 and ACTH 4–10, do not cause the release of corticosterone. These last offer the possibility that at least some of the direct effects of the full ACTH molecule can be determined using compounds which do not result in a simultaneous increase in corticosterone levels.

The use of ACTH 1–10 and ACTH 4–10 has demonstrated that increases in ACTH rather than corticosterone are responsible for the observed retardation of extinction of appetitive responding, active avoidance and passive avoidance. This conclusion is also supported by the fact that injections of corticosterone (which would increase corticosterone while decreasing ACTH) appear to speed up rather than retard extinction of both appetitive and avoidance tasks (Garrud, Gray & De Wied, 1974, also unpublished data from De Wied cited by them; see Leshner, 1977). The same appears to be true of the interactions of ACTH with frustration. Although the effects of ACTH 4–10 on the partial reinforcement extinction effect have not been reported, both ACTH 1–24 (which releases corticosterone) and ACTH 4–10 reduce the frustration effect seen when rats are transferred from acquisition to extinction of an appetitive response.

Chapter 7

1. Another way of looking at the double runway response is in terms of aversive motivation. We could suggest, for example, that the animals run faster in the second alley in order to escape from the first goal box in which reward was omitted. The idea that the first goal box is aversive also fits with the rats' behaviour in the first part of the runway. The partially rewarded rats run slower into the first goal box of the double runway, presumably in anticipation of the omission of reward (e.g. Ison, Daly & Glass, 1967). Genuine escape from reward omission is apparently demonstrated in an experiment by Adelman & Maatsch (1956). They provided rats with a way of jumping out from the goal box of a runway. During extinction of running in the runway the rats learned to jump out of the goal box faster than controls which were not being extinguished but which were rewarded with food for jumping out. Similarly, Wagner (1963) has shown that rats will learn to cross a hurdle to terminate a stimulus which has previously been paired with nonreward.

2. For reasons of economy and clarity Chapter 7 glosses over the reasons for assuming that the *omission* of significant stimuli can produce both unconditioned and conditioned states which have both motivational and releasing properties; and, in particular, the fact that the releasing properties of conditioned states may be different from those of unconditioned. The main concern within the chapter is that such internal states have sensory properties. Chapter 9 discusses in greater detail the evidence that the *presentation* of stimuli such as food and shock can elicit internal states which have the capacity not only to support learning and the performance of new responses but also to release species typical patterns of behaviour; and that previously neutral stimuli which predict the occurrence of such significant stimuli can also come to elicit central states. It will be shown that these conditioned states can have similar motivational properties to the unconditioned central states while having somewhat different (even diametrically opposed) releasing properties.

3. There are a number of procedural rules attached to the use of Sutherland's model, the critical one for our purposes being that the probability of an analyser being switched in or out takes longer to change than the strength with which a response becomes attached to any particular analyser.

The PREE is explained as follows. When animals are continuously rewarded, whatever analyser is switched in, will be reinforced. This both strengthens its connection with the response made and decreases the relative probability that other analysers will be switched in. Training will therefore develop considerable response strength to a limited number of analysers. In fact, even a modest amount of training should result in asymptotic strengthening of the connections. With partial reinforcement, no analyser will be consistently reinforced, and hence a large number of analysers will accrue some response strength. Since switching of analysers takes more experience than does changing the strength of response to a particular analyser, then many analysers of moderate strength will take longer to switch out than a few of high strength. It follows that the partially reinforced animals will take longer to extinguish than the continuously reinforced animals. Hence we have a PREE.

An important point at which this theory is tied to objective data is in its prediction that partially reinforced animals will learn more about the stimulus aspects of their environment than continuously reinforced animals (because they switch in more analysers). This prediction is not explicitly made by the alternative theories discussed in Chapter 7. Sutherland (1966) tested this prediction in a number of experiments in which animals learned two-choice discriminations under either continuous or partial reinforcement of the correct choice. The discriminations could be solved on the basis of any one of a number of classes of cue. For example, if thin horizontal stripes signal the correct choice and thick vertical stripes signal the incorrect choice, an animal need only attend to one of either width or orientation but not both. What the animal has actually learned can then be tested by giving it a choice where only one of the two stimulus dimensions is available (e.g. horizontal versus vertical stripes of the same, intermediate, thickness). With seven such stimulus dimensions available, Sutherland (1966) found that partially reinforced animals learned about approximately six dimensions while continuously reinforced animals learned about only one. Within the continuous group, the one particular dimension to which attention was directed varied from animal to animal.

4. A distinctive feature of Capaldi's (1967) theory is that it emphasises the order in which the animal receives particular sequences of N and R. For example, it predicts that, in the type of experiment described in Chapter 7 NNRNNRNNR etc. will produce a greater PREE than NRNRNR. This is because, in both cases, we have exactly three instances of reward and so equal resistance to extinction will have been built up which is attached in the first case to the stimulus NN and in the second case to the stimulus N. NN is between N and NNNNNNN (i.e. extinction) on the R–N continuum. Therefore, given the equal resistance to extinction attached to each, NN will produce greater generalisation to NNNNNNNNN than will N. There is considerable evidence supporting this type of prediction. The theory can also explain the occurrence of a PREE with very small numbers of acquisition trials (McCain, 1966, 1968; Bowen & McCain, 1967). With appropriate values for the slope of the generalisation curve one could predict a PREE in animals receiving as few as two trials.

5. Feldon *et al.* (1979) found no effect on the PREE in the start section of their alley in animals receiving drug both in acquisition and extinction. There was a reduction of the PREE in animals receiving saline in acquisition and drug in extinction. This cannot be due to an effect of the drug on processes such as toughening up or frustration since the drug was not present during the critical acquisition trials. In the absence of further evidence it seems reasonable to attribute this result to an interaction of stimulus properties of the drug state with stimulus after-effects of the type proposed by Capaldi. Thus, during acquisition the rats receive N paired with reward, but during extinction they receive (drug   N). Since N and (drug   N) are dissimilar, these rats will show less generalisation and hence less responding than those receiving N in extinction. This type of drug–after-effect interaction has been shown, although not with a 24-hour intertrial interval, in experiments carried out by Capaldi & Sparling (1971). They gave rats drug on only some days of acquisition so that for some rats (drug   N) was followed by reward and for others (saline   N) was followed by reward. With extinction under drug the (drug   N) rats were more resistant to extinction than (saline   N) rats, while the latter were

similar to continuously reinforced rats. With extinction under saline (saline N) rats were more resistant than (drug N) and the latter were similar to continuously reinforced rats.

6. This possibility is supported by results obtained by Brown & Wagner (1964). They carried out an experiment in which one group of rats were trained with partial punishment and continuous reward and a second group were trained with with partial omission of reward. Each of these groups were then divided into two further subgroups tested either with continuous punishment and continuous reward or with complete omission of reward (extinction). They found that partial punishment and partial reinforcement increased resistance to continuous punishment and to extinction respectively – that is to say they found the usual partial punishment and partial reinforcement effects. More importantly, they found that in the start section of their alley partial punishment in acquisition increased resistance to extinction and partial reinforcement increased resistance to continuous punishment. In other words there was a degree of cross-tolerance between punishment and omission of reward. However, this cross-tolerance accounted for less than half of the observed effects in the two standard groups. It seems reasonable to assume that this cross-tolerance represents non-associative toughening up and that the remaining, reinforcer-specific resistance could result from control of responding by stimulus after effects.

7. Ison & Pennes (1969), as was noted in Chapter 7, found symmetric state-dependency of the PREE. The effect of the drug was greatest in the start section and least in the goal section. Following the argument from Section 7.9, we may assume that the drug-sensitive component of the PREE in their experiment was due entirely to stimulus aftereffects compounded with drug state.

What of the drug-insensitive component of the PREE in their goal section? We may note that Ziff & Capaldi (1971) in a small trial, short intertrial interval experiment found a PREE only in the goal section and that this was also insensitive to the drug. We could account for all of the preceding as follows. With short intertrial intervals and small numbers of trials, stimulus after-effects are highly discriminable and are associated with the goal section of the alley. As number of trials or intertrial interval increases the exact pattern of N and R trials becomes less distinct to the animal and its influence on behaviour extends to other parts of the runway and can also become compounded with the stimulus properties of drug states. With sufficient acquisition, particularly with large rewards, unconditioned and then conditioned frustration develops. This leads to toughening up and, independently, to conditioning of running to stimuli of frustration. As with after-effects we presume that frustration is initially effective only in the goal segments of the runway.

Whatever the exact truth of the above, it seems reasonable to conclude that (a) the PREE is the result of a variety of different underlying control processes, each most effective under different conditions; and (b) the PREE depends on stimulus properties of conditioned frustration when a 24 hour intertrial interval is used and measurements are made in the goal box of a straight alley.

Chapter 8

1. Analysis of the various types of love is complicated by their interactive nature. In the early chapters we were able to concentrate on the emotional reaction of the individual and leave the eliciting stimulus to a large extent in the background. With love it can be a

matter of arbitrary choice which of two individuals we decide is the source of the stimuli, and it is the ongoing interaction of the individuals over time which is of central interest. This leads to some ambiguity in the term love (of whatever type). If we say that a parent loves their child, we are usually using the term in the sense of a trait rather than state – the parent may currently be *feeling* totally exasperated by the child. The experimental assessment of love as a state has not been developed to any great extent, particularly in non-humans.

In this context I would wish to distinguish love from lust (in the sense of sexual arousal, with no moral connotation). The specific physiological responses which accompany lust have been well described (Masters & Johnson, 1966); the eliciting stimuli for lust need involve no inter-individual interaction (magazine photographs are usually used as stimuli in experimental studies, e.g. Valins, 1967; Wenger, Averill & Smith, 1968); the biological determinants of sexual behaviour have been fairly well investigated (see, e.g. Hutchison, 1978); and finally, the teleonomy of specifically sexual behaviour seems straightforward.

It is particularly worth noting that lust, as identified by sexual behaviour, need have no connection with love, as reflected in pair bonding. For example, Hill, Rubin & Peplau (1976) found that whether dating couples would stay together for as much as two years was predicted by scores on Rubin's love scale but not by either copulation or cohabitation (or indeed by scores on a liking scale). Likewise other female primates will copulate (in the initial stages of heat) with a variety of males despite being part of a specific alpha male's harem.

Chapter 9

1. Blackman (pers. comm.) has suggested that this point is not clear cut since one could take the view that 'the "operant response" in a DRL schedule is the whole sequence of behaviour leading to a lever press (or as some would have it, the inter-response time). In this case, the frequency of this functional class may be decreased by the conditioned suppression procedure, thereby allowing another technical operant, namely "lever pressing" *tout court*, to emerge'.

2. Davison, Sheldon & Lobb (1980) present data which suggest 'that performance in the positive conditioned suppression procedure results from concurrent and multiple schedule interactions. The data further suggest that the production of either acceleration or suppression is dependent on adventitious and historical contingencies' (p.51). In Davison *et al.*'s experiment pigeons could peck either of two keys on each of which a variable interval schedule for keypecking was imposed. The stimulus signalling free food (or contingent food in some conditions) was presented on one of the keys. It is clear from their results that complex interactions can be obtained with concurrent schedules, and by implication that positive conditioned suppression as it is normally observed could result from an interaction between responses on the manipulandum and concurrent adventitious schedules imposed on responses not measured by the experimenter. However, further work is needed to show that such adventitious schedules are operative in the normal cases of positive conditioned suppression where the stimulus for free food is presented successively rather than concurrently with a 'no food' condition and particularly where the stimulus is more generally visible to the animal. In the pigeon case it is entirely possible that the stimulus for free food is invisible when it is responding on the baseline manipulandum. The effect of specifically linking the stimulus with a manipulandum is also unclear. Finally, given the results with autoshaping with an omission contingency, it should be tested how far pigeons and mammals may differ in the mechanisms of control of phenomena such as conditioned suppression.

3. This conclusion is reinforced by data from previous chapters. In Chapter 6 there is evidence for a diminution of emotional behaviour as avoidance conditioning proceeds; in particular with extreme examples of persistent avoidance, initial acquisition is followed (with no further experience of shock) by the development of stereotyped responding and a loss of peripheral emotional reactions (Solomon *et al.*, 1953). The data of Wynne & Solomon (1955) also imply that peripheral feedback, although not essential for the eventual acquisition of avoidance, makes an important contribution to normal acquisition.

Chapter 10

1. There is one discrepancy between the data presented by Ekman, Levenson & Friesen (1983) and that in Table 5.1: namely that Averill reported decreased heart rate in sadness and increased heart rate with mirth, whereas they report the reverse for sadness and happiness.

2. As an example of the extent to which such interactions are invoked even in models which presume that an emotion arises from some single central state see Buck (1983, particularly his Figure 9.2)

Chapter 11

1. The aquatic hypothesis is by no means conclusively proved. Nor is it supposed to exclude a major role in human evolution for the pressures provided by subsequent savannah living of the types discussed by Morris, Ardrey and others. The 'aquatic ape' if it existed would have been a precursor of australopithecines and hominids. Current theory probably favours a hunter–gatherer rather than killer ape adaptation as the driving force behind hominid evolution (Leakey, 1981). One advantage of the aquatic hypothesis is it describes an initial specific adaptation (to a seaside environment) which would account for the failure of other primates to take the same evolutionary path as humans given that they have been exposed over an immense period of time to virtually identical environmental contingencies.

2. Gray (1979) is somewhat dismissive of the idea that *defecation* in the mouse is a form of territorial marking and states that the increase in defecation over trials in this species 'does not clearly indicate anything very much'. However, it should be noted that one of Hall's basic justifications for the idea that defecation reflected fear was its reduction over time. An increase in defecation over time in the mouse does not necessarily mean that some of the defecation is not due to fear, but it does imply that some other factor is at work.

References

Adamec, R.E. & Stark-Adamec, C.I. 1983. Limbic control of aggression in the cat. *Progress in Neuropsychology and Biological Psychiatry*, **7**, 505–12

Adelman, H.M. & Maatsch, J.L. 1956. Learning and extinction based upon frustration, food reward and exploratory tendency. *Journal of Experimental Psychology*, **52**, 311–15

Ader, R. 1969. Adrenocortical function and the measurement of 'emotionality'. *Annals of the New York Academy of Sciences*, **159**, 791–805

Amsel, A. 1967. Partial reinforcement effects on vigor and persistence. In Spence, K.W. & Spence, J.T. (eds) *The psychology of learning and motivation*, Vol 1, Academic Press: New York

Amsel, A. & Roussel, J. 1952. Motivational properties of frustration. I. Effect on a running response of addition of frustration to the motivational complex. *Journal of Experimental Psychology*, **43**, 363–8

Andrew, R.J. 1963. Evolution of facial expression. *Science*, **142**, 1034–41

Andrew, R.J. 1965. The origins of facial expression. *Scientific American*, **213**, 88–94

Arnold, M.B. 1968. *The nature of emotion* Penguin

Arnold, M.B. 1970. *Feelings and emotions*. Academic Press: New York

Averill, J.R. 1969. Autonomic response patterns during sadness and mirth. *Psychophysiology*, **5**, 399–414

Ax, A.F. 1953. The physiological differentiation of fear and anger in humans. *Psychosomatic Medicine*, **15**, 433–42

Ax, A.F., Lloyd, R., Gorham, J.C., Lootens, A.M. & Robinson, R. 1978. Autonomic learning: a measure of motivation. *Motivation and Emotion*, **2**, 213–42

Azrin, N.H. 1967. Pain and aggression. *Psychology Today*, **1**, 25–33

Azrin, N.H., Hutchinson, R.R. & Hake, D.F. 1967. Attack, avoidance and escape reactions to aversive shock. *Journal of the Experimental Analysis of Behaviour*, **10**, 131–48

Bacon, F. 1900. *Advancement of Learning*. I.v.8, W.A. Wright (ed) 5th Edition, Clarendon Press:Oxford

Balakrishnan, M. & Alexander, K.M. 1976. Hormonal control of scent marking in the Indian musk shrew, *Suncus murinuus viridescens* (Blyth). *Hormones and Behaviour*, **7**, 431–9

Baltzer, V. & Weiskrantz, L. 1970. Negative and positive behavioural contrast in the same animals. *Nature*, **228**, 581–2

Bassili, J.N. 1979. Emotion recognition: the role of facial movement and the relative importance of upper and lower areas of the face. *Journal of Personality and Social Psychology*, **37**, 2049–58: cited by Krech *et al* (1982)

Beatty, D.A., Beatty, W.A., Bowman, R.E. & Gilchrist, J.C. 1970. The effects of ACTH, adrenalectomy and dexamethasone on the acquisition of an avoidance response in rats. *Physiology and Behaviour*, **5**, 939–44

Becker, G. 1969. Initial and habituated autonomic reactivity in the male and female rat. *Journal of Comparative and Physiological Psychology*, **69**, 459–64

Bermant, G. 1961a Response latencies of female rats during sexual intercourse. *Science*, **133**, 1771–3 cited by Carlson (1980)

Bermant, G. 1961b Regulation of sexual contact by female rats. Unpublished PhD. Dissertation, Harvard University, cited by Carlson (1980)

Bindra, D. 1969. A unified interpretation of emotion and motivation. *Annals of the New York Academy of Sciences*, **159**, 1071–83

Black, R.W. & Spence, K.W. 1965. Effects of intertrial reinforcement on resistance to extinction following extended training. *Journal of Experimental Psychology*, **70**, 559–63

Blackman, D.E. 1968. Conditioned suppression or acceleration as a function of behavioural baseline. *Journal of the Experimental Analysis of Behaviour*, **11**, 53–61

Blackman, D.E. 1983. On cognitive theories of animal learning: extrapolation from humans to animals. In Davey, G.C.L. (ed) *Animal models of human behaviour*. John Wiley, New York.

Blixt, S. & Ley, R. 1969. Force-contingent reinforcement in instrumental conditioning and extinction in children: a test of the frustration-drive hypothesis. *Journal of Comparative and Physiological Psychology*, **69**, 267–72

Bolles, R.C. 1970. Species-specific defense reactions and avoidance learning. *Psychological Review*, **71**, 32–48

Bolles, R.C. 1975. *Learning theory*. Holt, Rinehart, Winston: New York

Borda-Bossana, D., Elrick, H., Bernstein, L. & Atkinson, H. 1961. Effects of handling in the adrenalectomised rat treated with corticosterone. *Journal of Psychosomatic Research*, **5**, 206–10

Bouton, M.E. & Bolles, R.C. 1980. Conditioned fear assessed by freezing and the suppression of three different baselines. *Animal Learning and Behaviour*, **8**, 429–34

Bowen, J. & McCain, G. 1967. Occurrence of the partial reinforcement extinction effect after only one NRNR sequence of trials. *Psychonomic Science*, **9**, 15–6

Brady, J.V. 1975a. Conditioning and emotion. In Levi, L. (ed) *Emotions: their parameters and measurement*, Raven Press: New York

Brady, J.V. 1975b. Toward a behavioural biology of emotion. In Levi, L. (ed) *Emotions: their parameters and measurement*, Raven Press: New York, pp 17–46

Brannigan, C.R. & Humphries, D.A. 1972. Human non-verbal behaviour, a means of communication. In Blurton Jones, N. (ed) *Ethological studies on infant behaviour*, Cambridge University Press: Cambridge

Breland, K. & Breland, M. 1961. The misbehaviour of organisms. *American Psychologist*, **16**, 681–4

Bridges, K.M.B. 1931. *The social and emotional development of the preschool child*. Kegan Paul, Trench, Trubner

Broadhurst, P.L. 1957. Emotionality and the Yerkes–Dodson law. *Journal of Experimental Psychology*, **54**, 345–51

Broadhurst, P.L. 1960. Application of biometrical genetics to the inheritance of behaviour. In Eysenck, H.J. (ed) *Experiments in Personality*. Vol I: *Psychogenetics and psychopharmacology*, Routledge, Kegan, Paul

Brown, J.S. & Farber, I.E. 1951. Emotions conceptualised as intervening variables; with suggestions towards a theory of frustration. *Psychological Bulletin*, **48**, 465–95

Brown, P.L. & Jenkins, H.M. 1968. Autoshaping of the pigeons key peck. *Journal of the Experimental Analysis of Behaviour*, **11**, 1–8

Brown, R.T. & Wagner, A.R. 1964. Resistance to punishment and extinction following training with shock or nonreinforcement. *Journal of Experimental Psychology*, **68**, 503–7

Buchenauer, D., Luft, C. & Grauvogl, A. 1982. Investigation of the eliminative behaviour of piglets. *Applied Animal Ethology*, **9**, 153–64: abstract retrieved by DIALOG computer system

Buck, R. 1976. *Human emotion and motivation*. John Wiley, New York.

Buck, R. 1979. Individual differences in nonverbal sending accuracy and electrodermal responding: the externalising–internalising dimension. In Rosenthal, R. (ed) *Skill in nonverbal communication*, Oelgeschlager, Gunn & Hain: Cambridge, Massachusetts.

Buck, R. 1980. Nonverbal behaviour in the theory of emotion: the facial feedback hypothesis. *Journal of Personality and Social Psychology*, **38**, 811–24

Buck, R. 1983. Emotional development and emotional education. In Plutchik, R. & Kellerman, H. (eds) *Emotion: theory, research, and experience*. Vol 2. *Emotions in early development*, Academic Press: New York

Buck, R. 1985. Prime theory: an integrated view of emotion and motivation. *Psychological Review*, **92**, 389–413

Caldwell, D.F. 1962. Effects of adrenal demedullation on retention of a conditioned avoidance response in the mouse. *Journal of Comparative and Physiological Psychology*, **55**, 1079-81

Candland, D.K. 1977. The persistent problems of emotion. In Candland, D.K., Fell, J.P., Keen, E., Leshner, A.I., Plutchik, R. & Tarpy, R.M. (eds) *Emotion*. Brooks/Cole:Monterey, California

Candland, D.K. & Nagy, Z.M. 1969. The open field: some comparative data. *Annals of the New York Academy of Sciences*, **159**, 831–51

Cannon, W.B. 1927. The James-Lange theory of emotion. *American Journal of Psychology*, **39**, 106–124; reprinted in part in Arnold, M.B. 1968. (ed) *The nature of emotion*. Penguin

Cannon, W.B. 1936. *Bodily changes in pain, hunger, fear and rage*. Appleton-Century: New York

Cantrill, H. & Hunt, W.A. 1932. Emotional effects produced by the injection of adrenalin. *American Journal of Psychology*, **44**, 300–7

Capaldi, E.J. 1967. A sequential hypothesis of instrumental learning. In Spence, K.W. & Spence, K.T. (eds) *The psychology of learning and motivation*, Vol 1, Academic Press: New York

Capaldi, E.J. & Sparling, D.L. 1971. Amobarbital and the partial reinforcement effect in rats: isolating frustrative control over instrumental responding. *Journal of Comparative and Physiological Psychology*, **74**, 467–477

Carlson, N.R. 1980. *Physiology of behaviour*. 2nd Edition, Allyn and Bacon: Boston

Carroll, L. 1954. Through the looking glass and what Alice found there. In *Alice's adventures in Wonderland; Through the looking glass; and other writings*, Collins: London

Cervero, F. & Sharkey, K.A. 1985. More than just gut feelings about visceral sensation. *Trends in Neuroscience*, 8, 188–90

Champion, R.A., McCann, T.E., Ruffels, J.A. 1972. Frustration phenomena in paired-associate learning. *Journal of Experimental Psychology*, **95**, 123–34

Chen, J.S. & Amsel, A. 1977. Prolonged, unsignalled, inescapable shocks increase persistence in subsequent appetitive instrumental learning. *Animal Learning and Behaviour*, **5**, 377–85

Chevalier-Skolnikoff, S. 1973. Facial expression of emotion in non-human primates. In Ekman, P. (ed) *Darwin and facial expression*, Academic Press: New York

Chi, C.C. & Flynn, J.P. 1967. Neural pathways associated with the hypothalamically elicited attack behaviour of cats. *Science*, **171**, 703–6

Church, R.M. 1978. The internal clock. In Hulse, S.H., Fowler, H & Honig, W.K. (eds) *Cognitive processes in animal behaviour*, Lawrence Erlbaum: Hillsdale, New Jersey

Collins, R.L. 1966. What does the defecation score measure. *Proceedings of the 74th Annual Convention of the American Psychological Association*: abstract retrieved from the DIALOG computer system, pp. 147–8

Conan Doyle, A. 1928. Silver Blaze. In Conan Doyle, A. *The complete Sherlock Holmes stories*. John Murray Ltd: London

Coover, G.D., Goldman, L. & Levine, S. 1971. Plasma corticosterone increases produced by extinction of operant behaviour in rats. *Physiology and Behaviour*, **6**, 261–3

Coover, G.D., Ursin, H. & Levine, S. 1973. Plasma corticosterone levels during active avoidance learning in rats. *Journal of Comparative and Physiological Psychology*, **82**, 170–4

Crawford, M. & Masterson, F.A. 1978. Components of the flight response can reinforce bar press avoidance. *Journal of Experimental Psychology: Animal Behaviour Processes*, **4**, 144–51

Crespi, L.P. 1942. Quantitive variation of incentive and performance in the white rat. *American Journal of Psychology*, **55**, 467–517

Dana, C.L. 1921. The anatomic seat of the emotions: a discussion of the James-Lange theory. *Archives of Neurology and Psychiatry*, **6**, 634–9

Darwin, C. 1965. *The expression of the emotions in man and animals*. Univ. of Chicago Press, Chicago, Illinois.

Davison, M.C., Sheldon, L. & Lobb, B. 1980. Positive conditioned suppression: transfer of performance between contingent and non-contingent reinforcement situations. *Journal of the Experimental Analysis of Behaviour*, **33**, 51–7

Davitz, J.R. 1969. *The language of emotion*. Academic Press: New York

Dawkins, R. 1978. *The selfish gene*. Paladin/Granada: Frogmore, St. Albans

De Wied, D., van Delft, A.M.L., Gispen, W.H., Weijnen, J.A.W.M. & van Wimersma Greidanus, T.B. 1972. The role of pituitary–adrenal system hormones in active avoidance conditioning. In Levine, S. (ed) *Hormones and behaviour*, Academic Press: New York

Delgado, J.M.R. 1969. *Physical control of the mind*. Harper and Row: New York

Delgado, J.M.R. & Mir, D. 1969. Fragmental organisation of emotional behaviour in the monkey brain. *Annals of the New York Academy of Sciences*, **159**, 731–51

Denenberg, V.H. 1967. Stimulation in infancy, emotional reactivity and exploratory behaviour. In Glass, D.C. (ed) *Neurophysiology and emotion*, Rockefeller

Di Cara, L.V. & Weiss, J.M. 1966. Effect of heart-rate learning under curare on subsequent non-curarised avoidance learning. *Journal of Comparative and Physiological Psychology*, **69**, 368–74

Dickinson, A. 1980. *Contemporary animal learning theory*. Cambridge University Press: Cambridge

Ditkoff, G. & Ley, R. 1974. Effects of positive and negative force-contingent reinforcement on the frustration effect in humans. *Journal of Experimental Psychology*, **102**, 818–23

Duffy, E. 1941. An explanation of 'emotional' phenomena without the use of the concept 'emotion'. *Journal of General Psychology*, **25**, 283–93

Duffy, E. 1962. *Activation and behavior*. Wiley, New York

Efran, J.S. & Spangler, T.J. 1979. Why grown-ups cry: a two factor theory and evidence from the Miracle Worker. *Motivation and Emotion*, **3**, 63–72

Eibl-Eibesfeldt, I. 1971. *Love and hate*. Methuen: London

Ekman, P. 1982. *Emotion in the human face*. 2nd Edition, Cambridge University Press: Cambridge

Ekman, P. & Friesen, W.V. 1978. *Facial Action Coding System (FACS) A technique for measurement of facial action*. Palo Alto: Consulting Psychologists Press: cited by Redican (1982)

Ekman, P. & Friesen, W.V. 1982. Measuring facial movement with the facial action coding system. In Ekman, P. (ed) *Emotion in the human face*, 2nd edition, Cambridge University Press

Ekman, P. & Friesen, W.V. 1986. A new pan-cultural facial expression of emotion. *Motivation and Emotion*, **10**, 159–68

Ekman, P., Levenson, R.W. & Friesen, W.V. 1983. Autonomic nervous system activity distinguishes among emotions. *Science*, **221**, 1208–10

Ekman, P. & Oster, H. 1979. Facial expressions of emotion. *Annual Review of Psychology*, **30**, 527–54

Ekman, P., Roper, G. & Hager, J.C. 1980. Deliberate facial movement. *Child Development*, **51**, 886–91

Erdman, G. & Janke, W 1978. Interaction between physiological and cognitive determinants of emotions: experimental studies on Schachter's theory of emotions. *Biological Psychiatry*, **6**, 61–74

Estes, W.K. 1943. Discriminative conditioning: I. A discriminative property of conditioned anticipation. *Journal of Experimental Psychology*, **32**, 150–5

Estes, W.K. & Skinner, B.F. 1941. Some quantitative properties of anxiety. *Journal of Experimental Psychology*, **29**, 390–400

Eysenck, H.J. 1967. *The biological basis of personality*. Charles C. Thomas: Springfield, Illinois.

Fanselow, M.S. 1984. What is conditioned fear? *Trends in Neuroscience*, **7**, 460–2

Feldon, J., Guillamon, A., Gray, J.A., De Wit, H. & McNaughton, N. 1979. Sodium amylobarbitone and responses to nonreward. *Quarterly Journal of Experimental Psychology*, **31**, 19–50

Flynn, J.P. 1967. The neural basis of aggression in cats. In Glass, D.C. (ed) *Neurophysiology and emotion*, Rockefeller University Press: New York

Flynn, J.P. 1969. Neural aspects of attack behaviour in cats. *Annals of the New York Academy of Sciences*, **159**, 1008–12

Frankenhaeuser, M., Dunne, E. & Lundberg, V. 1976. Sex differences in sympathetic-adrenal medullary reactions induced by different stressors. *Psychopharmacology*, **47**,1–5

Frisby, J.P. 1979. *Seeing*. Oxford University Press

Funkenstein, D.H. 1955. The physiology of fear and anger. *Scientific American*, **192**, 74–80

Funkenstein, D.H., King, S.H. & Drolette, M. 1954. The dissection of anger during a laboratory stress-inducing situation. *Psychosomatic Medicine*, **16**, 404–13

Gallup, G.G. 1965. Aggression in rats as a function of frustrative non-reward in a straight alley. *Psychonomic Science*, **3**, 99–100

Gallup, G.G. & Hare, G.K. 1969. Activity following partially reinforced trials: evidence for a residual frustration effect due to conditioned frustration. *Psychonomic Science*, **16**, 41–42

Garrud, P., Gray, J.A. & De Wied, D. 1974. Pituitary–adrenal hormones and extinction of rewarded behavior in the rat. *Physiology and Behaviour*, **12**, 109–19

Gellhorn, E. 1960. Recent contributions to the physiology of the emotions. *Psychiatric Research Reports*, **12**

Gellhorn, E. 1964. Motion and emotion: the role of proprioception in the physiology and pathology of the emotions. *Psychological Review*, **71**, 457–472

George, F. & Johnson, L. (Eds) 1985. Purposive behaviour and teleological explanations. *Studies in Cybernetics:* **8**. Gordon & Breach: New York

Godbout, R.C., Ziff, D.R. & Capaldi, E.J. 1968. Effect of several reward exposure procedures on the small trial PREE. *Psychonomic Science*, **13**, 153–154

Goldstein, D., Fink, D. & Mettee, D.R. 1972. Cognition of arousal and actual arousal as determinants of emotion. *Journal of Personality and Social Psychology*, **21**, 41–51

Goldstein, M.L. 1968. Physiological theories of emotion: a critical review from the standpoint of behaviour theory. *Psychological Bulletin*, **69**, 23–40

Gould, J.L. 1982. *Ethology*. Norton: New York

Gray, J.A. 1968. The physiological basis of personality. *Advancement of Science*, **24**, 293–305

Gray, J.A. 1970. The psychophysiological basis of introversion–extraversion. *Behaviour Research and Therapy*, **8**, 249–265

Gray, J.A. 1971a. *The psychology of fear and stress*. Weidenfeld and Nicholson: London

Gray, J.A. 1971b. Effect of ACTH on extinction of rewarded behaviour is blocked by previous administration of ACTH. *Nature*, **229**, 52–54

Gray, J.A. 1975. *Elements of a two-process theory of learning*. Academic Press: London

Gray, J.A. 1977. Drug effects on fear and frustration: possible limbic site of action of minor tranquillisers. In Iversen, L.L., Iversen, S.D. & Snyder, S.H. (eds) *Handbook of Psychopharmacology*. Vol. 8, Plenum Press: New York

Gray, J.A. 1979. Emotionality in male and female rodents: a reply to Archer. *British Journal of Psychology*, **70**, 425–40

Gray, J.A. 1982. *The neuropsychology of anxiety: an enquiry into the functions of the septo-hippocampal system*. Oxford University Press: New York

Gray, J.A. 1987. *Fear and stress* (2nd edition) Cambridge University Press: Cambridge

Gray, J.A. & Dudderidge, H. 1971. Sodium amylobarbitone, the partial reinforcement effect, and the frustration effect in the double runway. *Neuropharmacology*, **10**, 217–22

Gray, J.A., Holt, L. & McNaughton, N. 1983. Clinical implications of the experimental pharmacology of the benzodiazepines. In Costa, E. (ed) *The benzodiazepines: from molecular biology to clinical practice*, Raven Press: New York

Gray, J.A., Mayes, A.R. & Wilson, M. 1971. A barbiturate-like effect of adrencorticortropic hormone on the partial reinforcement acquisition and extinction effects. *Neuropharmacology*, **10**, 223–30

Hager, J. 1982. Asymmetries in facial expression. In Ekman, P. (ed) *Emotion in the human face*, 2nd edition, Cambridge University Press

Halgren. E. 1982. Mental phenomena induced by stimulation in the limbic system. *Human Neurobiology*, **1**, 251–60

Hall, C.S. 1934a. Drive and emotionality: factors associated with adjustment in the rat. *Journal of Comparative Psychology*, **17**, 89–108

Hall, C.S. 1934b. Emotional behaviour in the rat: I. Defecation and urination as measures of individual differences in emotionality. *Journal of Comparative Psychology*, **18**, 385–403

Hall, C.S. 1941. Temperament: a survey of animal studies. *Psychological Bulletin*, **38**, 909–43

Halpern, J. & Poon, L. 1971. Human partial reinforcement extinction effects: an information-processing development from Capaldi's sequential theory. *Journal of Experimental Psychology Monographs*, 207–227

Hanson, H.M. 1959. Effects of discriminative training on stimulus generalisation. *Journal of Experimental Psychology*, **58**, 321–34

Hardy, A. 1960. Was man more aquatic in the past? *New Scientist*, **7**, 642–5: reprinted in Morgan (1982)

Harlow, H.F. & Harlow, M.K. 1962. Social deprivation in monkeys. *Scientific American*, **207**, 136–46

Harlow, H.F. & Stagner, R. 1933. Psychology of feelings and emotion. I. Theory of emotions. *Psychological Review*, **40**, 184–94

Hilgard, E.R., Atkinson, R.C. & Atkinson, R.L. 1971. *Introduction to psychology* (5th Edition), Harcourt Brace Jovanovich Inc.

Hill, C.T., Rubin, Z. & Peplau, A. 1976. Breakups before marriage: the end of 103 affairs. *Journal of Social Issues*, **32**, 147–67: cited by Krech et al (1982)

Hinde, R.A. 1966. *Animal behaviour*. McGraw-Hill: New York

Hinde, R.A. 1970. *Animal behaviour*. (Second Edition), McGraw-Hill Kogakusha: Tokyo

Hinde, R.A. 1982. *Ethology*. Fontana Paperbacks

Hofer, M.A. 1972. Physiological and behavioural processes in early maternal deprivation. In Porter, R. & Knight, J. (eds) *Physiology, emotion and psychosomatic illness*, CIBA symposium No: 8 (new series), Elsevier

Hofer, M.A. 1983. On the relationship between attachment and separation processes in infancy. In Plutchik, R. & Kellerman, H. (eds) *Emotion: theory, research and experience*. Vol 2. *Emotions in early development*, Academic Press: New York, pp 199–219

Hofer, M.A., Wolff, C.T., Friedman, S.B. & Mason, J.W. 1972*a*. A psychoendocrine study of bereavement: Part I. 17-hydroxycorticosteroid excretion rates and patterns following the death of their children from leukemia. *Psychosomatic Medicine*, **34**, 481–91

Hofer, M.A., Wolff, C.T., Friedman, S.B. & Mason, J.W. 1972*b*. A psychoendocrine study of bereavement: Part II. Observations on the process of mourning in relation to adrenocortical function. *Psychosomatic Medicine*, **34**, 492–502

Hohman, G.W. 1966. Some effects of spinal cord lesions on experienced emotional feelings. *Psychophysiology*, **3**, 143–5

Hoyenga, K.B. & Hoyenga, K.T. 1984. *Motivational explanations of behaviour*. Brooks/Cole: Monterey, California.

Hume, D. 1969. *A treatise on human nature*. Penguin Books

Hunt, H.F. & Otis, L.S. 1953. Conditioned and unconditioned emotional defecation in the rat. *Journal of Comparative and Physiological Psychology*, **46**, 378–82

Hutchison, J.B. (ed) 1978. *Biological determinants of sexual behaviour*. John Wiley & Sons: Chichester

Iacono, R.P. & Nashold, B.S. 1982. Mental and behavioural effects of brain stem and hypothalamic stimulation in man. *Human Neurobiology*, **1**, 273–80

Isaacson, R.L., Hutt, M.L. & Blum, M.L. 1965. *Psychology: the science of behaviour*. Harper and Row: New York

Ison, J.R., Daly, H.B. & Glass, D.H. 1967. Amobarbital sodium and effects of reward and nonreward in the Amsel double runway. *Psychological Reports*, **20**, 491–6

Ison, J.R. & Pennes, L. 1969. Interaction of amobarbital sodium and reinforcement schedule in determining resistance to extinction of an instrumental running response. *Journal of Comparative and Physiological Psychology*, **68**, 215–9

Izard, C.E. 1979. (ed) *Emotions in personality and psychopathology*. Plenum Press: New York

Izard, C.E. & Buechler, S. 1979. Emotion expressions and personality integration in infancy. In Izard, C.E. (ed) *Emotion in personality and psychopathology*, Plenum Press: New York

James, W. 1884. What is an emotion? *Mind* (1884) **9**, 188–205; reprinted in Arnold, M.B. 1968. (ed) *The nature of emotion*, Penguin Modern Psychology

Jasnos, T.M. & Hakmiller, K.L. 1975. Some effects of lesion level and emotional cues on affective expression in spinal cord patients. *Psychological Reports* **37**, 859–70

Jenkins, H.M. & Moore, B.R. 1973. The form of the autoshaped response with food or water reinforcers. *Journal of the Experimental Analysis of Behaviour*, **20**, 163–81

Jenkins, W.O. & Stanley, J.C. 1950. Partial reinforcement. A review and critique. *Psychological Bulletin*, **47**, 193–234

Johansson, G., Collins, A. & Collins, V.P. 1983. Male and female psychoneuroendocrine response to examination stress: a case report. *Motivation and Emotion*, **7**, 1–9

Johnston, T.D. 1981. Contrasting approaches to a theory of learning. *Behavioural and Brain Sciences*, **4**, 125–73

Kamin, L.J., Brimer, C.J. & Black, A.H. 1963. Conditioned suppression as a monitor of fear of the CS in the course of avoidance training. *Journal of Comparative and Physiological Psychology*, **56**, 497–501

Kandel, E.R. & Schwartz, J.H. 1985. *Principles of neural science*. Second Edition. Elsevier: New York

Kaufman, I.C. & Rosenblum, L.A. 1969. Effects of separation from mother on the emotional behaviour of infant monkeys. *Annals of the New York Academy of Sciences*, **159**, 681–95

Kelly, J.F. & Hake, D.F. 1970. An extinction-induced increase in an aggressive response with humans. *Journal of the Experimental Analysis of Behaviour*, **14**, 153–64

Kimble, G.A. 1961. *Hilgard and Marquis's conditioning and learning*. 2nd edition, Appleton-Century-Crofts: New York

Kleiman, D.G. 1975. The effects of exposure to conspecific urine on urine-marking in male and female degus (*Octodon degus*). *Behavioural Biology*, **14**, 519–26

Klinnert, M.D., Campos, J.J., Sorce, J.F., Emde, R.N. & Svejda, M. 1983. Emotions as behaviour regulators. In Plutchik, R. & Kellerman, H. (eds) *Emotion: theory, research, and experience*. Vol 2. *Emotions in early development*, Academic Press: New York

Konishi, M. 1971. Ethology and neurobiology. *American Scientist*, **59**, 56–63

Krebs, J.R. Stephens, D.W. & Sutherland, W.J. 1983. Perspectives in optimal foraging. In Clark, G.A. & Brush, A.H. (eds) *Perspectives in ornithology*, Cambridge University Press

Krech, D., Crutchfield, R.S., Livson, N., Wilson, W.A. & Parducci, A. 1982. *Elements of psychology*. 4th Edition, Alfred Knopf: New York

Lader, M., Tyrer, P. 1975. Vegetative system and emotion. In Levi, L. (ed) *Emotions: their parameters and measurement*, Raven Press: New York

Land, E.H. 1959. Experiments in colour vision. *Scientific American*, **200**, 84–9

Lanzetta, J.T., Cartwright–Smith, J. & Kleck, R.E. 1976. Effects of nonverbal dissimulation on emotional experience and autonomic arousal. *Journal of Personality and Social Psychology*, **33**, 354–70

Latane, B. & Schachter, S. 1962. Adrenaline and avoidance learning. *Journal of Comparative and Physiological Psychology*, **55**, 369–72

Leakey, R.E. 1981. *The making of mankind*. Michael Joseph Ltd: London

Leshner, A.I. 1977. Hormones and emotion. In Candland, D.K., Fell, J.P., Keen, E., Leshner, A.I., Plutchik, R. & Tarpy, R.M., *Emotion*. Brooks/Cole: Monterey, California.

Levi, L. 1965. The urinary output of adrenaline and noradrenaline during pleasant and unpleasant emotional states. *Psychosomatic Medicine*, **27**, 80–5

Levine, S. 1971. Stress and behaviour. *Scientific American*, **224**, 26–31

Levine, S., Haltmeyer, G.C., Karas, G.G. & Denenberg, V.H. 1967. Physiological and behavioural effects of infantile stimulation. *Physiology and Behaviour*, **2**, 55–9

Levine, S. & Jones, L.E. 1965. Adrenocorticotropic hormone (ACTH) and passive avoidance learning. *Journal of Comparative and Physiological Psychology*, **59**, 357–60

Levine, S. & Soliday, S. 1962. The effect of adrenal demedullation on the acquisition of conditioned avoidance responses. *Journal of Comparative and Physiological Psychology*, **55**, 214–16

Lewis, D.J. 1960. Partial reinforcement: a selective review of the literature since 1950. *Psychological Bulletin*, **57**, 1–28

Leyhausen, P. 1956. Verhaltenstudien bei Katzen. *Zeitschrift fur Tierpsychologie* Beiheft, 2, cited by Fentress, J.C. (1978) Conflict and context in sexual behaviour. In Hutchison, J.B. (ed) *Biological determinants of sexual behaviour*. Wiley: Chichester

Llinas, R.R. & Simpson, J.I. 1981. Cerebellar control of movement. In Towe, A.L. & Luschei, E.S. (eds) *Handbook of behavioural neurobiology*. Vol. 5: *Motor coordination*, Plenum Press: New York

Lorenz, K. 1952. Die Entwicklung der vergleichenden Verhaltensforschung in den letzten 12 Jahren. *Verhandlung der Deutsche Zoologische Gesellschaft*, 36–58: cited by Eibl-Eibesfeldt (1971)

Lyons, W. 1980. *Emotion*. Cambridge Studies in Philosophy Series, Cambridge University Press,

Mackintosh, N.J. 1974. *The psychology of animal learning*. Academic Press: London

Malatesta, C.Z. 1981. Infant emotion and the vocal affect lexicon. *Motivation and Emotion*, **5**, 1–23

Mandler, G. 1962. Emotion. In Newcombe, T.M. (ed) *New directions in psychology*. Holt, Rinehart Winston:New York, pp. 269–343

Mandler, G. 1975. *Mind and emotion*. Wiley

Mandler, G. 1984. *Mind and body*. Norton: New York

Mandler, G. & Kahn, M. 1960. Discrimination of changes in heart rate: two unsuccessful attempts. *Journal of the Experimental Analysis of Behaviour*, **3**, 21–5

Maslach, C. 1979. The emotional consequences of arousal without reason. In Izard, C.E. (ed) *Emotion in personality and psychopathology*, Plenum Press: New York

Mason, J.W. 1975. Emotion as reflected in patterns of endocrine integration. In Levi, L. (ed) *Emotions: their parameters and measurement*, Raven Press: New York

Masters, W.H. & Johnson, V.E. 1966. *Human sexual response*. Little Brown: Boston

Masterson, F.A. & Crawford, M. 1982. The defense motivation system: a theory of avoidance behaviour. *Behavioural and Brain Sciences*, **5**, 661–75

McCain, G. 1966. Partial reinforcement effects following a small number of acquisition trials. *Psychonomic Monograph Supplements*, **1**, No 12, 251–69

McCain, G. 1968. The partial reinforcement effect after minimal acquisition: single pellet reward. *Psychonomic Science*, **13**, 151–2

McFarland, D.J. 1971. *Feedback mechanisms in animal behaviour*. Academic Press: London

McFarland, D.J. & McGonigle, B. 1967. Frustration tolerance and incidental learning as determinants of extinction. *Nature*, **214**, 531–2

McKelligott, J. 1959. Autonomic function and affective state in spinal cord injury. Unpublished doctoral dissertation, University of California at Los Angeles; cited by Jasnos & Hakmiller, 1975

McNamara, J. & Houston, A. 1980. The application of statistical decision theory to animal behaviour. *Journal of Theoretical Biology*, **85**, 673–90

McNaughton, N. & Mason, S.T. 1980. The neuropsychology and neuropharmacology of the dorsal ascending noradrenergic bundle – a review. *Progress in Neurobiology*, **14**, 157–219

Millenson, J.R. & De Villiers, P.A. 1972. Motivational properties of conditioned anxiety. In Gilbert, R.M. & Millenson, J.R. (eds) *Reinforcement: behavioural analyses*, Academic Press: New York

Millenson, J.R. & Leslie, J.C. 1974. The conditioned emotional response (CER) as a baseline for the study of anti-anxiety drugs. *Neuropharmacology*, **13**, 1–9

Millenson, J.R. & Leslie, J.C. 1979. *Principles of behaviour analysis*. 2nd edition, Macmillan: New York

Miller, N.E. 1948. Studies of fear as an acquirable drive: I. Fear as motivation and fear as reinforcement in the learning of new responses. *Journal of Experimental Psychology*, **38**, 89–101

Miller, N.E. 1976. Learning, stress and psychosomatic symptoms. *Acta Neurobiologia Experimentalis*, **36**, 141–56

Miller, R.E. & Ogawa, N. 1962. The effect of adrenocorticotropic hormone (ACTH) on avoidance conditioning in the adrenalectomised rat. *Journal of Comparative and Physiological Psychology*, **55**, 211–3

Mineka, S. & Gino, A. 1980. Dissociation between conditioned emotional response and extended avoidance performance. *Learning and Motivation*, **11**, 476–502

Monod, J. 1974. *Chance and necessity*. Fontana Books/William Collins, Glasgow

Morgan, E. 1982. *The aquatic ape*. Souvenir Press, London

Morris, D. 1967. *The naked ape*. Dell Publishing Co: New York

Moyer, K.E. 1958a. Effect of adrenalectomy on anxiety motivated behaviour. *Journal of Genetic Psychology*, **92**, 11–6

Moyer, K.E. 1958b. Effect of adrenalectomy on emotional elimination. *Journal of Genetic Psychology*, **92**, 17–21

Moyer, K.E. & Bunnell, B.N. 1959. Effect of adrenal demedullation on avoidance responses in the rat. *Journal of Comparative and Physiological Psychology*, **52**, 215–6

Moyer, K.E. & Bunnell, B.N. 1960a. Effect of adrenal demedullation on the startle response of the rat. *Journal of Genetic Psychology*, **97**, 341–4

Moyer, K.E. & Bunnell, B.N. 1960b. Effect of adrenal demedullation, operative stress and noise stress on emotional elimination. *Journal of Genetic Psychology*, **96**, 375–82

Neftel, K.A., Adler, R.H., Kappeli, L., Rossi, M., Dolder, M., Kaser, H.E., Bruggesser, H.H. & Vorkauf, H. 1982. Stage fright in musicians: a model illustrating the effect of beta blockers. *Psychosomatic Medicine*, **44**, 461–9

Neisser, U. 1967. *Cognitive psychology*. Appleton-Century-Crofts: New York

Nelson, T.O. 1971. Extinction, delay and partial reinforcement effects in paired associate learning. *Cognitive Psychology*, **2**, 212–28

Nicholson, J.N. & Gray, J.A. 1971. Behavioural contrast and peak shift in children. *British Journal of Psychology*, **62**, 367–73

Nicholson, J.N. & Gray, J.A. 1972. Peak shift, behavioural contrast and stimulus generalisation as related to personality and development in children. *British Journal of Psychology*, **63**, 47–62

Nietzsche, F. 1961. Der Antichrist. Reprinted in Podach, E.F. (ed) *Friedrich Nietzsche's Werke des Zusammenbruchs*, Wolfgang Rother: Heidelberg

Notterman, J.M. 1959. Force emission during bar pressing. *Journal of Experimental Psychology*, **58**, 341–7

O'Keefe, J. & Nadel, L. 1978. *The hippocampus as a cognitive map*. Oxford University Press

Occam, Gulielmus de 1957. : Quodlibeta, V, Q.i. In Boehner, P. (ed) *Ockham: Philosophical Writings*, Nelson: Edinburgh

Orr, S.P. & Lanzetta, J.T. 1984. Extinction of an emotional response in the presence of facial expression of emotion. *Motivation and Emotion*, **8**, 55–66

Orwin, W. 1969. Escape and avoidance learning in extremely neurotic and extremely stable subjects. *British Journal of Social and Clinical Psychology*, **8**, 362–74

Overton, D.A. 1966. State-dependent learning produced by depressant and atropine-like drugs. *Psychopharmacology*, **10**, 6–31

Panksepp, J. 1982. Toward a general psychobiological theory of emotions. *Behavioural and Brain Sciences*, **5**, 407–20

Papez. J.W. 1937. A proposed mechanism of emotion. *Archives of Neurological Psychiatry*, **38**, 725–43: reprinted in part in Arnold (1968)

Pare, W.P. 1969. The effect of adrenalectomy, adrenal demedullation and adrenaline on the aversive threshold in the rat. *Annals of the New York Academy of Sciences*, **159**, 869–79

Pascal, B. 1925. Pensées. In *Oeuvres de Blaise Pascal*. Vol 13 (ed) L. Brunschvicg. 3rd edition, Libraire Hachette: Paris

Paul, C. & Havlena, J. 1962. Maze learning and open field behaviour of adrenalectomised rats. *Journal of Psychosomatic Research*, **6**, 153–6

Pearce, J.M. & Hall, G.H. 1980. A model for Pavlovian learning: variations in the effectiveness of conditioned but not of unconditioned stimuli. *Psychological Review*, **87**, 532–52

Pittendrigh, C.S. 1958. Adaptation, natural selection and behaviour. In A. Roe & G.G. Simpson (eds) *Behaviour and Evolution*. Yale University Press; cited by Staddon, J.E.R. (1983)

Plutchik, R. 1983. Emotions in early development: a psychoevolutionary approach. In Plutchik, R. & Kellerman, H. (eds) *Emotion: theory, research and experience*. Vol 2. *Emotions in early development*, Academic Press: New York, pp. 221–257

Plutchik, R. & Ax, A.F. 1967. A critique of determinants of emotional state by Schachter and Singer (1962). *Psychophysiology*, **4**, 79–82

Pribram, K.H. 1970. Feelings as monitors. In Arnold M.B. (ed) *Feelings and emotions*. Academic Press

Redican, W.K. 1982. An evolutionary perspective on human facial displays. In Ekman, P. (ed) *Emotion in the human face*. 2nd Edition, Cambridge University Press: Cambridge

Renfrew, J.W. & Hutchinson, R.R. 1983. The motivation of aggression. In Satinoff, E and Teitelbaum, P. (eds) *Handbook of behavioural neurobiology*. Vol. 6: *Motivation*, Plenum Press

Rescorla, R.A. 1978. Some implications of a cognitive perspective on Pavlovian conditioning. In Hulse, S.H., Fowler, H. & Honig, W.K. (eds) *Cognitive processes in animal behaviour*, Lawrence Erlbaum: Hillsdale, New Jersey

Rescorla, R.A., Lo Lordo, V.M. 1965. Inhibition of avoidance behaviour. *Journal of Comparative and Physiological Psychology*, **59**, 406–12

Rescorla, R.A. & Solomon, R.L. 1967. Two-process learning theory: relationships between Pavlovian conditioning and instrumental learning. *Psychological Review*, **74**, 151–82

Ridgers, A. & Leslie, J.C. 1975. Autoshaping and omission training in the rat. Paper read to Experimental Analysis of Behaviour Group, Exeter, England (1975): cited by Millenson & Leslie (1979)

Riskind, J.H. & Gotay, C.C. 1982. Physical posture: could it have regulatory or feedback effects on motivation? *Motivation and Emotion*, **6**, 273–98

Roberts, D.C.S. & Fibiger, H.C. 1977. Evidence for interaction between central noradrenergic neurones and adrenal hormones in learning and memory. *Pharmacology, Biochemistry and Behaviour*, **7**, 191–4

Roberts, E. 1984a. GABA neurons in the mammalian central nervous system: model for a minimal basic neural. *Neuroscience Letters*, **47**, 195–200

Roberts, E. 1984b. The inhibited nervous system: roles of GABAergic neurons. *Neuropharmacology*, **23**, 863–4

Roberts, R.J. & Weerts, T.C. 1982. Cardiovascular responding during anger and fear imagery. *Psychological Reports*, **50**, 219–30

Rorty, A.O. 1980. *Explaining emotions*. University of California Press: Berkely

Rosenzweig, M.R. & Leiman, A.L. 1982. *Physiological psychology*. Heath and Co., Lexington, Mass.

Royce, J.R. 1977. On the construct validity of open field measures. *Psychological Bulletin*, **84**, 1098–106

Russell, P.A. 1973. Open field defecation in rats: relationships with body weight and basal defecation level. *British Journal of Psychology*, **64**, 109–14

Ryan, T.J. & Watson, P. 1968. Frustrative nonreward theory applied to childrens behaviour. *Psychological Bulletin*, **69**, 111–25

Salmon, P. & Gray, J.A. 1985a. Comparison of the effects of propranolol and chlordiazepoxide on timing behaviour in the rat. *Psychopharmacology*, **87**, 219–24

Salmon, P. & Gray, J.A. 1985b. Opposing acute and chronic behavioural effects of a beta-blocker, propranolol, in the rat. *Psychopharmacology*, **86**, 480–6

Salmon, P. & Gray, J.A. 1986. Effects of propranolol on conditioned suppression, discriminated punishment and discriminated non-reward in the rat. *Psychopharmacology*, **88**, 252–7

Schachter, S. 1957. Pain, fear and anger in hypertensives and normotensives: a psychophysiologic study. *Psychosomatic Medicine*, **19**, 17–29

Schachter, S. 1971. *Emotion, obesity and crime*. Academic Press: New York

Schachter, S. 1980. Non-psychological explanations of behaviour. In Festinger, L. (ed) *Retrospections on social psychology*, Oxford University Press

Schachter, S. & Singer, J.E. 1962. Cognitive, social and physiological determinants of emotional state. *Psychological Review*, **69**, 379–99

Schachter, S. & Wheeler, L. 1962. Epinephrine, chlorpromazine and amusement. *Journal of Abnormal and Social Psychology*, **65**, 121–8

Schandry, R. 1981. Heart beat perception and emotional experience. *Psychophysiology*, **18**, 483–8

Schnore, M.M. 1959. Individual patterns of physiological activity as a function of task differences and degree of arousal. *Journal of Experimental Psychology*, **58**, 117–28

Schwartz, G.E., Weinberger, D.A. & Singer, J.A. 1981. Cardiovascular differentiation of happiness, sadness, anger and fear following images and exercise. *Psychosomatic Medicine*, **43**, 343–64

Scott, J.P. 1980. The function of emotions in behavioural systems: a systems theory analysis. In Plutchik, R. & Kellerman, H. (eds) *Emotion: theory, research and experience*. Vol. 1: *Theories of emotion*, Academic Press: New York

Shaffer, L.F. 1947. Fear and courage in aerial combat. *Journal of Consulting Psychology*, **11**, 137–43, cited by Hilgard *et al.* 1971

Shakespeare, W. (undated) Macbeth. In Craig, W.J. (ed) *The complete works of William Shakespeare*. Clarendon Press: Oxford (The Oxford Shakespeare)

Sheffield, F.D. & Temmer, H.W. 1950. Relative resistance to extinction of escape training and avoidance training. *Journal of Experimental Psychology*, **40**, 287–98

Shelley, P.B. 1903. *Poems*. Blackie and Sons: London

Shettleworth, S.J. 1973. Food reinforcement and the organisation of behaviour in golden hamsters. In Hinde, R.A. & Stevenson-Hinde, J. (eds) *Constraints on learning*, Academic Press: London

Shettleworth, S.J. 1978. Reinforcement and the organisation of behaviour in golden hamsters: punishment of three action patterns. *Learning and Motivation*, **9**, 99–123

Shettleworth, S.J. & Juergensen, M.R. 1980. Reinforcement and organisation of behaviour in golden hamsters: brain stem reinforcement for seven action patterns. *Journal of Experimental Psychology*, **6**, 352–75

Sirota, A.D., Schwartz, G.E. & Shapiro, D. 1974. Voluntary control of human heart rate: effect on reaction to aversive stimulation. *Journal of Abnormal Psychology*, **83**, 261–7

Sirota, A.D., Schwartz, G.E. & Shapiro, D. 1976. Voluntary control of human heart rate: effect on reaction to aversive stimulation: a replication and extension. *Journal of Abnormal Psychology*, **85**, 473–7

Slucki, H., Adam, G., Porter, R.W. 1965. Operant discrimination of an interoceptive stimulus in rhesus monkeys. *Journal of the Experimental Analysis of Behaviour*, **8**, 405–14

Smith, C.A., McHugo, G.T. & Lanzetta, J.T. 1986. The facial patterning of posed and imagery induced expressions of emotions by expressive and nonexpressive posers. *Motivation and Emotion*, **10**, 133–57

Sokolov, E.N. 1960. Neuronal models and the orienting reflex. In Brazier, M. (ed) *The central nervous system and behaviour*

Solomon R.C. 1977. The logic of emotion. *Nous*, **11**: cited by Lyons (1980)

Solomon, R.L., Kamin, L.J. & Wynne, L.C. 1953. Traumatic avoidance learning: the outcome of several extinction procedures with dogs. *Journal of Abnormal Psychology*, **48**, 291–302

Solomon, R.L. & Turner, L.H. 1962. Discriminative classical conditioning in dogs paralysed by curare can later control discriminative avoidance responses in the normal state. *Psychological Review*, **69**, 202–19

Staddon, J.E.R. 1983. *Adaptive behavior and learning*. Cambridge University Press

Stanners, R.F., Coulter, M., Sweet, A.W. & Murphy, P. 1979. The pupillary response as an indicator of arousal and cognition. *Motivation and Emotion*, **3**, 319–40

Starr, M.D. & Mineka, S. 1977. Determinants of fear over the course of avoidance learning. *Learning and Motivation*, **8**, 332–50

Stouffer, S.A., Lumsdaine, A.A., Lumsdaine, M.H., Williams, R.M., Smith, M.B., Janis, I.L., Star, S.A. & Cottrell, L.S. 1949. *Studies in social psychology in world war II*: Vol 2. *The american soldier: combat and its aftermath*. Princeton; cited by Broadhurst, P.L. (1969) page 37

Strongman, K.T. 1978. *The psychology of emotion.* 2nd edition, Wiley: Chichester

Suomi, S.J., Mineka, S. & Harlow, H.F. 1983. Social separation in monkeys as viewed from several motivational perspectives. In Satinoff, E. and Teitelbaum, P (eds) *Handbook of behavioural neurobiology.* Vol. 6: *Motivation*, Plenum Press: New York

Sutherland, N.S. 1964. The learning of discrimination by animals. *Endeavour*, **23**, 148–52

Sutherland, N.S. 1966. Partial reinforcement and breadth of learning. *Journal of Experimental Psychology*, **18**, 289–301

Taylor, J. 1956. Drive theory and manifest anxiety. *Psychological Bulletin*, **53**, 303–20

Terrace, H.S. 1966. Stimulus control. In Honig, W.K. (ed) *Operant behaviour: areas of research and application*, Appleton-Century-Crofts: New York

Timberlake, W. & Grant, D.L. 1975. Autoshaping in rats to the presentation of another rat predicting food. *Science*, **190**, 690–2

Tobach, E. & Schneirla, T.C. 1962. Eliminative responses in mice and rats and the problem of 'emotionality'. In Bliss, E.L. (ed) *Roots of behaviour*, Harper

Towe, A.L. & Luschei, E.S. 1981. Preface. In Towe, A.L. & Luschei, E.S. (eds) *Handbook of behavioural neurobiology.* Vol. 5: *Motor coordination*, Plenum Press: New York

Truax, S.R. 1983. Active search, mediation and the manipulation of cue dimensions: emotion attribution in the false-feedback paradigm. *Motivation and Emotion*, 7, 41–60

Valins, S. 1967. Emotionality and information concerning internal reactions. *Journal of Personality and Social Psychology*, **6**, 458–63

Valins, S. & Ray, A.A. 1967. Effects of cognitive desensitisation on avoidance behaviour. *Journal of Personality and Social Psychology*, **7**, 345–50

Van Toller, C. & Tarpy, R.M. 1972. Effect of cold stress on the performance of immunosympathectomised mice. *Physiology and Behaviour*, **8**, 515–7

Van Toller, C. & Tarpy, R.M. 1974. Immunosympathectomy and avoidance behaviour. *Psychological Bulletin*, **81**, 132–7

Wagner, A.R. 1959. The role of reinforcement and non-reinforcement in the 'apparent frustration effect'. *Journal of Experimental Psychology*, **57**, 130–6

Wagner, A.R. 1963. Conditioned frustration as a learned drive. *Journal of Experimental Psychology*, **66**, 142–8

Waller, M.B. & Waller, P.F. 1963. The effects of unavoidable shock on a multiple schedule having an avoidance component. *Journal of the Experimental Analysis of Behaviour*, **6**, 29–37

Wallin, G. & Fagius, J. 1986. The sympathetic nervous system in man – aspects derived from microelectrode recordings. *Trends in Neurosciences*, **9**, 63–6

Walsh, R.N. & Cummins, R.A. 1976. The open field test: a critical review. *Psychological Bulletin*, **83**, 482–504

Watson, J.B. 1924. *Behaviorism.* W.W. Norton & Co: New York

Watson, J.B. 1929. *Psychology from the standpoint of a behaviourist.* 3rd edition, Rensel, Lippincott: Philadelphia: cited by Strongman (1978)

Weisman, R.G. & Litner, J.S. 1972. The role of Pavlovian events in avoidance training. In Boakes, R.A. & Halliday, M.S. (eds) *Inhibition and learning*, Academic Press: New York

Wenger, M.A., Averill, J.R. & Smith, D.B. 1968. Autonomic activity during sexual arousal. *Psychophysiology*, **4**, 468–78

Wenzel, B.M. 1968. Behavioural studies of immunosympathectomised mice. *Journal of Comparative and Physiological Psychology*, **66**, 354–62

Wenzel, B.M. & Jeffrey, D.W. 1967. The effect of immunosympathectomy on behaviour of mice in aversive situations. *Physiology and Behaviour*, **2**, 193–201

Wenzel, B.M., Nagle, B. 1965. The effects of immunosympathectomy on behavior in mice. *Experimental Neurology*, **12**, 399–410

Whimbey, A.E. & Denenberg, V.H. 1967. Two independent behavioural dimensions in open field performance. *Journal of Comparative and Physiological Psychology*, **63**, 500–4

Wickelgren, W.A, 1979. *Cognitive Psychology*. Prentice Hall: Englewood Cliffs, N.J.

Williams, D.R. & Williams, H. 1969. Automaintainance in the pigeon: sustained pecking despite contingent nonreinforcement. *Journal of the Experimental Analysis of Behaviour*, **12**, 511–20

Wynne, L.C. & Solomon, R.L. 1955. Traumatic avoidance learning: acquisition and extinction in dogs deprived of normal peripheral autonomic function. *Genetic Psychology Monographs*, **52**, 241–84

Ziff, D.R. & Capaldi, E.J. 1971. Amytal and the small trial partial reinforcement effect: stimulus properties of early trial nonrewards. *Journal of Experimental Psychology*, **87**, 263–9

Zimbardo, P.G., Ebbesen, E.B. & Maslach, C. 1977. *Influencing attitudes and changing behaviour*. Addison Wesley: Reading, Massachusetts

Zucker, I. 1983. Motivation, biological clocks and temporal organisation of behaviour. In Satinoff, E. and Teitelbaum, P. (eds) *Handbook of behavioural neurobiology*. Vol. 6. *Motivation*, Plenum Press: New York

Index

Subject index